FE

A

The Household Environment
and Chronic Illness

The Household Environment and Chronic Illness

GUIDELINES FOR CONSTRUCTING AND MAINTAINING A LESS POLLUTED RESIDENCE

Edited by

GUY O. PFEIFFER, M.D.
Link Clinic
Mattoon, Illinois

and

CASIMIR M. NIKEL, F.A.C.H.A.
Health Ecology Systems Co.
Clovis, New Mexico

With a Foreword by

Richard Mackarness, M.B., B.S., D.P.M.
Psychiatrist in Charge
Clinical Ecology Research Unit
Basingstoke District Hospital
Hampshire, England

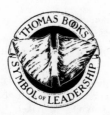

CHARLES C THOMAS • PUBLISHER
Springfield • Illinois • U.S.A.

Published and Distributed Throughout the World by
CHARLES C THOMAS ● PUBLISHER
Bannerstone House
301-327 East Lawrence Avenue, Springfield, Illinois, U.S.A.

© *1980, by* CHARLES C THOMAS ● PUBLISHER
ISBN 0-398-03961-5
Library of Congress Catalog Card Number: 79-9493

With THOMAS BOOKS *careful attention is given to all details of*
manufacturing and design. It is the Publisher's desire to present books that
are satisfactory as to their physical qualities and artistic possibilities and
appropriate for their particular use. THOMAS BOOKS *will be true to those*
laws of quality that assure a good name and good will.

Printed in the United States of America
V-00-2

Library of Congress Cataloging in Publication Data
Pfeiffer, Guy O.
  The household environment and chronic illness.

  Includes index.
  1. Housing and health. 2. Dwellings — Environmental
engineering.   3. Environmentally induced diseases.
4. Allergy. I. Pfeiffer, Guy O. II. Nikel,
Casimir M.
RA770.H64   613.5   79-9493
ISBN 0-398-03961-5

CONTRIBUTORS

JOHN W. ARGABRITE, M.D.
Argabrite Allergy Clinic, Watertown, South Dakota; Professor, South Dakota University, Vermillion, South Dakota

LEE ROY BYRD, M.D.
Private practice, Port Arthur, Texas; Fellow, American Association of Clinical Immunology & Allergy; Fellow, American Occupational Medical Association

SIDNEY J. HEIMAN
Board Chairman of Intertherm Inc., St. Louis, Missouri

JOHN G. MACLENNAN, M.D.
Hamilton General Hospital, Hamilton, Ontario, Canada

H. READ MINER
President of Air De-Pollution Inc., Decatur, Illinois

CASIMIR M. NIKEL, F.A.C.H.
Health Ecology Systems Co.; Former Administrator, Deaconess Hospital, Cleveland, Ohio; Fellow, American College of Hospital Administrators; Associate Fellow, Society for Clinical Ecology

GUY O. PFEIFFER, M.D.
Private practice, Mattoon, Illinois; Mattoon Memorial Hospital; Link Clinic of Mattoon, Illinois

THERON G. RANDOLPH, M.D.
Private practice, Chicago, Illinois; Professor, Northwestern University, Evanston, Illinois

FRANCIS V. SILVER
Diplomat, American Academy of Environmental Engineers; Fellow, Royal Society for Health

D.B. WARNOCK, LL.B., J.D.
Private practice, Edwardsville, Illinois; Member, Society for Clinical Ecology

FOREWORD

In 1951 Doctor A. R. P. Walker, Director of the Human Biochemistry Research Unit of the South African Medical Research Council, carried out a general health survey. This survey included the major causes of death on 73,000 people who were living in south India. The ten causes of death turned out to be infectious illnesses, and if the individual survived any of these diseases, such a patient, if fifty years old, had a 14.5 percent chance of reaching seventy.

Emigration to South Africa was common at that time from south India, where poverty was a great factor. Walker was able to compare his data with similar information about Indians who had moved to Johannesburg and who were living in comfortable urban surroundings. Here the main causes of death were coronary heart disease, strokes, cancer, and diabetes of those aged fifty or over of which only 9 percent reached the age of seventy.

Walker's studies indicated that at middle age, the prosperous immigrant, urban Indians in South Africa had a reduced life expectancy compared with their economically deprived friends and relatives back home. Many other similar studies carried out on comparable population groups have all shown similar differences. This suggests that living in towns reduces life expectancy and changes the pattern of disease.

Why should this be? Many different theories have been advanced, but all agree in putting some of the blame on changed environment.

Bringing the problem of environment-related disease to our own doorstep in Britain and America, what do we find? — a very similar story, if we compare indigenous people now with their forbears of a century ago. Famous nineteenth century British clinicians, such as Lord Lister and Sir William Osler, who were skilled observers, did not see many of the diseases

vii

that are so common today. In 1893 Osler could find only five cases of angina pectoris in over 8,000 patients. He reckoned a medical student lucky if he saw one case of coronary artery disease during his entire training period. A medical student today in London or New York could see ten cases in one week.

Since the industrial revolution began drawing people into the cities, concentrating them in polluted surroundings, and feeding them factory-produced chemicalized food, not only has the life expectancy of the middle-aged person remained static, but the morbidity of these persons has increased. Such persons now suffer a new and wider spectrum of diseases; one person in three has an allergy that is severe enough to take him to the doctor, and one in ten has migraine or high blood pressure. Heart disease affects one in three. One-half of the population is a stone* overweight, and one-fourth of the population is definitely obese. Tooth decay is rampant. One family in five has a mentally disturbed member, and one woman in nine spends some time under psychiatric care. Something has gone wrong. What is the medical profession doing about it? Not very much, I am sorry to say.

In America more and more general practitioners have stopped making housecalls. They are phasing themselves out of overall responsibility for the patient. They are increasingly becoming specialists, so that if a person becomes ill, it is necessary for him to decide which part of him is out of order and then try to find the appropriate specialist — not an easy task when feeling sick all over.

In Britain general practice of medicine has itself been turned into a specialty, which is so unspecialized that all but the simplest problems are referred to the hospitals. This leaves the G.P. practicing with little more than a ballpoint pen and a prescription pad. And under these circumstances the drug companies are having a field day.

John Fry, a well-known British G.P. practicing at Beckenham in Kent, who was one of the prime movers in founding the Royal College Of General Practice, describes in his book,

---

Stone is an official term designating British unit of weight, equal to 14 pounds.

Common Diseases — Their Nature, Incidence and Care, the three shocks awaiting the newly hospital-qualified physician entering general practice. Shock number one is "the rude awakening that comes to the physician on entering primary care and practice — to be faced with a mass of apparently unrecognized, undefinable and unfamiliar emotional disorders" (1). Shock number two is that these disorders cannot be categorized neatly like blood diseases, gastric ulcers, or bone fractures. Many of these disorders cannot be diagnosed or labelled with any accuracy at all. Shock number three comes with the realisation that cure is almost impossible in these conditions.

By "emotional disorders" Doctor Fry means those that manifest themselves as disturbances of thought, feeling, and behaviour. These are traditionally the province of the psychiatrist, but as there are not nearly enough psychiatrists to tackle such a large problem, the G.P. usually has to try to deal with the emotional disorders himself. This is an impossible task when he has no idea as to how they arise. And when you add to what Fry calls emotional illness the host of other new and equally mysterious illnesses that affect the body rather than behaviour, it is small wonder that doctors now have the highest suicide rate of any profession or trade.

All this uncertainty and confusion in modern medical practice leaves the patient with no one effective to turn to, unless his illness happens to be traumatic, infective, or recognizably pathologic, such as anaemia or myxoedema, which are correctible with medication. Fortunately into this void has stepped in a new breed of physician — namely, the clinical ecologist.

Clinical ecology is the study of effects in people who are maladapted to inhalants, contactants and ingestants in their physical environment. These effects may involve several systems of the body at the same time. They present themselves as polysymptomatic syndromes that tend to be dismissed as functional or hysterical after standard tests for pathology have proved negative. Frequently, ecologic health effects, or more correctly health impairments, are recognized clinical entities with pathological changes of unknown cause. Conversely, clinical ecology seeks to relate these idiopathic effects to the individual's environment.

Clinical ecology is really nothing new. It is a return to sound, whole-person medicine as it was practiced before the explosion of specialisation, which reduced the patient to a pigeon-holed assortment of unrelated parts. Actually, recognition of environmental or ecological factors in disease goes back a long way. The Chinese emperor, Shen Nung in 3000 B.C., forbade pregnant women to eat fish, chicken, and horsemeat because it was believed that these foods caused ulceration of the skin, which they certainly can if the individual happens to be allergic to them. Egyptian medical records indicate the death of King Menes in 2641 B.C. from a hornet sting, which is the result of an environmental impact. The great Galen (139-55 B.C., the best-remembered Greek physician in Rome) had taken the Hippocratic tradition of careful observation of environmental causes for illness to Italy. He described classical migraine as related to foods and sneezing as occurring in the presence of certain plants.

During the past two years in Britain, clinical ecology has been gaining favorable attention. This is partly due to the efforts of Doctor Randolph and the Society for Clinical Ecology, which was organized in 1965 at Las Vegas, Nevada. Some of the general practitioners under socialized medicine are also beginning to recognize the ecology of food and chemical susceptibility. An example of this was a lead article in *The Lancet* on February 3, 1979. It concluded, "Clearly food intolerance can produce widespread symptoms in susceptible individuals and many patients with troublesome and hitherto intractable symptoms can be now helped." If food allergy is now accepted, allergy to chemicals of the indoor environment must next engage the serious attention of doctors.

It is encouraging to introduce this book, which has been skillfully put together by Guy Pfeiffer and Casimir Nikel. It is not only timely, but it is a vital contribution to the management of ecological illness, which is incited by the indoor environmental conditions. To emphasize my regard for this book, I shall keep it on the desk in my consulting room, and I shall recommend it to every patient I see.

RICHARD MACKARNESS

REFERENCE

1. Fry, John: *Common Diseases — Their Nature, Incidence and Care.* Lancaster, England, Medical & Technical Publications Limited, 1974.

PREFACE

CHEMICALS that aggravate chronic illness may be found in the atmosphere, within the home, or in ingested substances. They are usually identified through a trial-and-error investigation. The individual who learns to observe his activities and surroundings before experiencing acute episodes of illness will often locate the causative agents. He will soon recognize that he experiences illness only when exposed to these agents or the gases that they release.

This volume presents practical ideas that may aid the individual who has chronic illness to obtain a less contaminated environment, to experience less pain, to develop a sense of well-being, and to live a more normal life.

The contributing authors are practical individuals who have learned to observe chronic illness and to determine the causes of the illness by an elimination procedure. No speculative theories are presented therefore, only clinically observed cause-and-effect relationships are discussed in this book.

The coeditors wish to thank the contributing authors, their patient families and their office assistants for their efforts. Other practical clinicians have shared their experiences with the contributing authors; we thank them for their part in the important field of preventive medicine.

GUY O. PFEIFFER

INTRODUCTION

To the first-time reader on the subject of environmental health care, this book may seem to be unusual. Its authors would agree with this viewpoint, principally because it is a pioneering effort in a fledgling medical specialty. This fledgling specialty is termed Clinical Ecology, which deals with the environmental etiology and therapy of diseases.

Clinical ecology established its formal organizational structure (Society for Clinical Ecology) less than fifteen years ago. Its preceding research and practice, however, were broad and profound enough to give it maturity at its formal inception. The mature judgment of clinical ecologists postulates that some human diseases are related to "the environment associated with air, water, food, drugs, and our habitat." Extensive research and clinical experience has been achieved in the area of air, water, food, and drugs. The human habitat has received, however, scant attention. It is an awareness of this neglect to the habitat as an impacting ecologic factor in human diseases that has impelled the authors of this book to produce it.

A new entity, such as clinical ecology, generally produces a newly formed nomenclature and an aggregation of new concepts. It seems, therefore, imperative that a glossary be provided with such a work as this book. Such words as allergies, clinical, chemical, ecologic, outgassing, susceptibility, hypersensitivity, etc., seem to be self-explanatory. Within the framework of clinical ecology in various combinations, these words, however, introduce new concepts. In some discussion situations these words have been given a specialized meaning. "Hypersensitivity" is one such example. For these reasons a glossary of selected terms that are conceptually significant has been produced.

Normally readers make reference to the glossary when they encounter a strange term during the reading of the text. In the instance of this book, wherein the Glossary basically defines concepts instead of terms (words), it is suggested that the reader of this book review the Glossary before proceeding with the text. Hopefully, this unorthodox perusal will result in a more perceptive comprehension of the text material.

The readers will find it helpful to note the following:

1. An italicized word indicates that it is defined in the Glossary.
2. Asterisks, daggers, etc. following a term indicates a footnote explanation.
3. A bracketed number, such as (1), following a quotation indicates a reference at the end of the chapter.

During the planning stage of this book, it became evident that the ecology of housing is in a high state of ferment. The coeditors were compelled to admit that some of the material and concepts might be obsolete before conclusion of the work. This was an unavoidable risk. The benefits to be derived in serving as guidelines toward a poorly illuminated goal seemed worthy of the risk. Therefore within the vortex of swirling progress, this book is presented with a hope for constructive benefit to its potentially studious readers.

CASIMIR M. NIKEL

CONTENTS

xviii   *The Household Environment and Chronic Illness*

The Household Environment
and Chronic Illness

Chapter 1

WHY AN ECOLOGIC HOUSE

THERON G. RANDOLPH

THE uninitiated might wonder, "Why a book on the ecology of housing?" After all, a house is a house, mainly for the purpose of providing shelter against either excessive cold (including wind and rain) or excessive heat. What is the difference between houses?

This difference can be stated simply. The house in which one lives, including its location, often makes the difference between a person's being healthy, happy, productive, and competitive or being chronically ill, depressed, unproductive, and noncompetitive. Moreover, housing impinges on a person's health and welfare by various degrees and combinations of these pluses and minuses. The degree of this impingement varies greatly between given persons, as well as between different houses. Especially involved is the individual's susceptibility to given environmental exposures, by the extent to which one's housing either insulates him against exposure or accentuates his contact with inciting environmental factors.

The ecology of housing is not only for the person who already knows that he has one or more *allergies*, for anyone is capable of becoming sensitive to a wide variety of environmental materials. Furthermore, he may or may not know when or if this might have occurred. A few extreme examples will be cited to illustrate this problem, with the understanding that lesser extremes are more commonplace. One person developed a severe allergy to horses shortly after moving into a remodeled old coach house. Seven members of one family became ill with various allergic manifestations within a year after moving into a do-it-yourself new home in which creosote-treated sleepers had been used as floor supports in combination with hot water radiant floor heating. Many other examples of allergic reactions to biological and chemical environmental exposures

3

could be given.

In order to better prepare the reader for using this book, background material leading up to this subject — the hygiene of housing — will be reviewed briefly. This will include a concise presentation of *clinical ecology*, or allergy in a wider frame of reference than it is usually considered, and how this illness is usually manifested. The housing environment capable of impinging on susceptible persons will be considered in its biologic and chemical aspects. Special emphasis will be placed on the latter, or so-called *chemical susceptibility* problem. This is becoming increasingly important in relation to medical problems associated with housing as earlier, largely inert building materials are being replaced by relatively more volatile and active synthetically derived substitutes.

DEFICIENCIES OF HUMAN NEEDS IN HOUSING

As primitive humans extended their range from warmer to colder climates, shortages of essential needs soon developed. Presumably the first deficiency occurred in housing as the available supply of suitable caves in a given area was quickly occupied. This probably led to overcrowding and possibly to smoke inhalation in at least certain less desirable parts of a cave. No doubt this deficiency and, perhaps, air contamination led to the construction of substitute housing. The type of building material used apparently varied from place to place, depending on the availability of supplies.

The next shortage of basic human needs apparently occurred in clothing and food supplies. Initially as a human group moved into a given area, an abundance of large game provided food as well as furs and hides for building materials and clothing. As long as abundant supplies of large animals persisted, carnivorous man apparently led a nomadic existence following such herds. According to one theory, the colonization of the Western Hemisphere by the initial immigrants from Asia advanced across the Americas in concentric waves extending from the Bering beachhead to Patagonia.

The availability of water and air apparently posed no major

problems for early nomadic man, other than that of water-borne infections and air pollution associated with poorly ventilated housing. But as population pressures increased in relation to the disappearance of available large animals and as deficiencies of housing, clothing, and food could no longer be met simply by wandering, domestication of animals apparently met these needs for several more millenia. Then gradually the nomadic herdsman life-style apparently was succeeded by permanent homes, and an agricultural and fishing society developed. Because of their ease of storage and high nutritional value, cereal grains were largely used for food during winter months while perishable food became the staple of the warmer months.

Housing, as we know it now, became concentrated in villages and, later, in urban communities, coincident with the onset of the industrial revolution. This began in Europe about 200 years ago and in America about a century later. Although complications of an industrial society affected the quality of all basic human needs (such as air, water, food, clothing and shelter) none were more adversely affected than housing, which is the subject of this book.

Indeed, industrial development in housing during the last century has been so rapid that we now have old-fashioned, relatively good housing and new-fashioned, relatively poor housing existing side by side. We also have excellent old houses, except for the fact that they may have been contaminated by exterminator residues, as well as good new housing, as far as its basic features are concerned, made relatively uninhabitable for some individuals by a poor selection of utilities and furnishings. These points will be developed in detail in later chapters.

A major point to emphasize at this time is that what constitutes "good housing" is a highly individualized matter. A good house for one person may be a poor one for another, depending on the existence of given allergies and the presence of inciting exposures. This brings us to a consideration of what is meant by allergies. This relatively new point of view is also best presented in its historical perspective.

THE HISTORY OF CLINICAL ALLERGY

Although the existence of acute allergic reactions, attributable to intermittent contacts, date back to antiquity, the big problem, with respect to housing, is concerned with chronic effects resulting from day-in and day-out or cumulative exposures. Within the framework of clinical allergy, intermittent exposures are far more apt to be suspected than chronic or cumulative exposures — even though an equal degree of individual susceptibility may exist to both. The latter tends to give rise to a self-perpetuating addictive type of response initially, in which each oft-repeated exposure to a given substance is followed by a relatively stimulatory effect. One simply remains stimulated and relatively free of symptoms as long as such specific exposures are encountered frequently and regularly. For instance, one does not ordinarily suspect the home gas utilities when exposed on a daily basis, whereas he may become acutely ill temporarily after first returning home from a vacation, until such a susceptible person again adjusts or adapts to the inhalation of such hydrocarbons.

In keeping with this basic difference between widely spaced and cumulative exposures, allergies to rarely eaten foods were recognized 2000 years ago, whereas allergic reactions to such commonly eaten foods as eggs were first described in 1912, and the most widely distributed common food, corn, was not identified until 1944. There was also a very retarded recognition of the man-made environmental *chemical exposures*.

Although *clinical manifestations* resulting from the common combustion products and derivatives of gas, oil, and coal were first described by several allergists at the mid-century point (1-4), the first comprehensive report of this problem did not occur until 1961 (5).

With respect to housing, the subject of the chemical susceptibility problem is still not commonly recognized for what it actually is — namely, the most common demonstrable cause of adverse reactions to given homes. Although aspects of this subject will be covered in subsequent chapters, at this point it is sufficient to say that the chemical susceptibility problem and housing are closely related.

Also, the more synthetic or chemically derived materials of gas, oil, coal, and conifer origin entering the basic construction, utilities, and furnishings of homes, the more likely the problem of chemical susceptibility is apt to exist in the occupants, and the more difficult it may be to identify the major causes of chronic ills. Indeed, many homes are so heavily chemically contaminated that, as a result of cumulative exposures and chronic reactions, the clearest way to recognize the existence of this problem is to remove a person to an ecologically controlled surrounding. The essentially addictive chronic responses are first accentuated, as in the case of *withdrawal effects*, before they subside. Following an extended exposure to the ecologically controlled surroundings, the patient arrives at a symptom-free condition. Then when such a relatively symptom-free person returns to his home, he tends to experience an acute diagnostically significant reaction (6,7). Similar test reactions are sometimes observed after returning from vacations. It is under these circumstances that a chemically susceptible individual might suspect the household environment as the cause of his chronic ailments.

CLINICAL MANIFESTATIONS

The previously mentioned clinical allergy often presents initially such stimulatory manifestations as hyperactivity, restless legs, obesity, alcoholism, and aggressive manic behavior. The environmental causes of such illnesses, due to frequently repeated exposure to foods or environmental chemical exposures, are usually not suspected. Sooner or later, these stimulatory manifestations, however, give way to physical and/or mental symptoms.

The various levels of the withdrawal syndromes consist of the well-known localized allergies, chronic upper or lower respiratory symptoms, hives, eczema, gastrointestinal, and genitourinary illnesses. The less well-known systemic allergies consist of fatigue, headache, musculoskeletal aches and pains, and a wide range of cardiovascular symptoms. These may be followed by lesser mental and behavior symptoms, such as "brain-fag" or more advanced depression and related psychotic disturbances.

Importantly, the responsible cause or causes of these chronic manifestations are rarely correctly identified (8).

There is a wide range of chronic allergic-ecologic illnesses of unsuspected cause. Housing, including basically structural features, along with equipment, furnishings, and supplies of homes is a major contributor to the origin and perpetuation of these illnesses (6-8).

INDIVIDUAL SUSCEPTIBILITY AND TOXICOLOGY

Some environmental exposures associated with housing are truly allergens in the same way that pollens, molds, dusts, insects, and animal danders are capable of inducing and perpetuating allergies in an immunological sense. Others, especially environmental chemical exposures that are known to be toxic in greater concentrations, are also responsible for chronic allergic manifestations in the trace amounts usually encountered. Clinical ecology — a wider framework than allergy in a limited immunologic sense — is particularly concerned with these chemical environmental exposures. These chemical exposures are especially important in housing. Not only must housing be designed with the specific allergic diagnosis of a patient in mind, but sound housing, in which environmental exposures described in this book are to be minimized or avoided, is important in the prophylaxis of chronic allergic disease.

BIBLIOGRAPHY

1. Coca, A.F.: *Familial Nonreaginic Food Allergy*, Second edition. Springfield, Thomas, 1945.
2. Lockey, S.D.: Allergic reactions due to FD&C dyes as coloring and identifying agents in various medications. *Bull Lancaster Gen Hosp*, September, 1948.
3. Wittich, F.W.: Respiratory tract allergic effects from chemical air pollution. *Arch Indust Hygiene*, 2:329, 1950.
4. Randolph, T.G.: Sensitivity to petroleum, including its derivatives and antecedents. *J Lab & Clin Med*, 40:931, 1952.
5. Randolph, T.G.: *Human Ecology and Susceptibility to the Chemical Environment*. Springfield, Thomas, 1962.
6. Randolph, T.G.: Specific adaptation. *Ann Allergy*, 40:333-345, May, 1978.
7. Randolph, T.G.: Stimulatory and withdrawal levels and the alternation of

allergic manifestations. In Dickey, L.D. (Ed.): *Clinical Ecology.* Springfield, Thomas, 1976.

8. Randolph, T.G.: The history of ecologic mental illness. In Frazier, C.A. (Ed.): *Annu Rev of Allergy, 1973.* Flushing, Med Exam, 1974.

Chapter 2

THE QUESTION OF GEOGRAPHY

JOHN G. MACLENNAN

A CERTAIN number of people in the general
population suffer from sensitivity to the chemical environment.
This is an illness that requires that certain measures of avoidance be taken to enable such persons to remain physically and
mentally well. When the specific causes of their sickness have
been identified, measures are devised to avoid exposures. Sometimes adequate avoidance within the existing environment is
impossible. To maintain good health the individual under
such circumstances is advised to seek out a new location for his
home. The new environment will not only assist in clearing up
the existing symptoms, but it will also delay or prevent the
future development of *ecologic disease.*

Ecologic disease can be compared to an iceberg. The visible
portion can be equated with the existing manifestations of the
disease that requires immediate diagnosis and treatment. The
submerged portion represents the latent, on-going, and developing future disease. A preventative approach to such illness is
superior to the treatment of symptoms after the disease surfaces.
To utilize disease prevention, it is important to follow ecologic
principles in locating the home. When there are strong allergies other than common chemical susceptibility among the
members of a family, relocation of residence might delay or
prevent further development of disease.

It is imperative under the foregoing circumstances to become
thoroughly familiar with all the different sensitivities possessed
by the chemically susceptible person. That requires a detailed
study of all the different causes of contactual, inhalant, and
food reactions. It is as important to know about all sensitivities
as it is to know about the common chemical exposures. It is
very important to treat all the patient's reactions, because if one
area of sensitivity is left untreated, then a successful solution of

10

the problem will not be achieved.

The urgency with which remedial measures require initiation depends upon the existing degree of chemical susceptibility. The extremely susceptible person will require immediate diagnostic and treatment measures. Those measures will include avoidance of the offending exposures, and/or injections, and/or geographic relocation of the home. In the instance where a minor to moderate degree of susceptibility is present, a program of avoidance of chemical exposures may suffice to solve the problem. After a suitable trial period if avoidance of exposures is not successful, then relocation of residence is carried out.

Economic factors must be considered in reaching a decision regarding relocation of one's home. If economic resources prevent relocation to a suburban or rural location, then a selective move within the urban area must be made, preferably on a temporary basis. The proposed new site should have the highest possible elevation on the windward* side of the community and away from all large industry that produces offending emissions. When economic considerations are not too restrictive, the conditions for geographic relocation of the home are much more flexible and permit a more ideal long-term solution of the problem.

There are certain important general conditions that must be considered when any geographical location of the home for a chemically susceptible person is being made. A careful, detailed assessment of the environs is made within a radius of ten miles of the proposed area for the new home. Downwind drift of chemical emissions will affect sensitive persons who live several miles from the source. This is particularly true in certain localities, i.e. in areas with high humidity, the air pollution tends to cling to the ground. If low valleylike land topography exists, it may funnel pollution for many miles.

Climatic factors are of unusual importance. These factors include uniformity of weather, frequency of storms, prevailing winds, extremes of temperature, annual precipitation, and prevailing humidity. The topography of the land may have an

---

*"Windward" means upstream of the prevailing wind currents from the location of the polluting source.

important bearing on movement of air and dissipation of offending chemical fumes, odors, and smokes. The survey should assess the prevailing land use relative to forestation, agriculture, industry, railroads, airports, traffic arteries, refuse landfills, and sewage disposal facilities.

A significant hazard might be presented by terrestial or airborne herbicides and pesticides. Farm crop and forest-spraying operations with such chemicals must be avoided. The new home should definitely be situated on the windward side of all these possible exposures.

When a residential survey is indicating the site for the new home, be sure to consider the highest point of land and avoid low-lying ground. Gas- and oil-heated real estate subdivisions should be avoided. Subdivisions of all-electric homes should be sought out if at all possible. At the least, the home should be an all-electric home. Conditions conducive to atmospheric inversions are particularly hazardous to the chemically susceptible person. These conditions may develop soon after you move into your new home if the real estate subdivision is new. It may be advisable, therefore, to locate on a quiet street in a built-up part of the community. A section about ten years old may be the most desirable one.

New neighborhoods present special hazards, such as freshly surfaced blacktop streets, or use of herbicides and pesticides, which might be used in establishing new lawns and new landscaping. Later-built homes also contain many synthetic materials that are frequently harmful to the chemically susceptible person.

Conversely, older homes have some handicaps. The older heating systems are generally less efficient. Loose construction may allow for dust infiltration. Aged wood may require termite spraying. All these may prove troublesome.

The home of the chemically susceptible person should be in reasonably close proximity to the place of employment. This will provide maximum avoidance of traffic fumes encountered enroute to and from work. An automobile air conditioner is an essential piece of equipment in reducing the impact of *ambient* air pollution exposures. When using an auto air conditioner, it is important that the outside-air intake is closed. Stopping behind other cars at intersections creates a special hazard if the outside-air intake is opened. Under such circumstances, the exhaust from the cars ahead that are waiting for traffic light changes can be sucked in and pollute air in the auto of the chemically sensitive and thereby precipitate a reaction. Use of ambient chemical-extracting air purifiers can reinforce the safety for the chemically sensitive auto passenger.

If a decision must be made to live in an apartment complex, then an electrohydronic or steam-heated type is preferred. In order to avoid exposure to chemical emissions from chimneys, rooftop air coolers, tar roofing materials, and exhaust ventilation, the living suite should be located on the windward side of the building and preferably several floors down from the top. Care should also be taken to locate well away from stair wells, elevator shafts, and nearby incinerators. The outside-air intake for the heating and cooling systems should be located on the windward side of the building. The higher floors of the building are the best location when the building is electrically heated.

A location near the shoreline where onshore breezes prevail can be beneficial in providing uncontaminated air, provided the body of water is large enough to allow dissipation of any contamination from passing water carriers.

When an extreme degree of chemical susceptibility is present, a rural or aquatic location may become a necessity. A large acreage on a waterfront is desirable in order to locate one's home strategically with regard to the ecologic exposures already mentioned, such as various inhalants made up of dust, pollens, mold spores, fumes, odors, and smokes.

Intensively farmed areas should be avoided. A woodlot located on the windward side may act as a protective barrier to airborne pollutants. If the person is sensitive to animal dander, then avoidance of feedlots, stockyards, and corrals becomes doubly important.

A dividend associated with a rural homesite is the ready access to clean water, which can be derived from a drilled deep well or from an artesian spring. Another dividend can be derived from suitable acreage — it can satisfy the need for organic vegetables, fresh fruits, uncontaminated meats and poultry, plus unpolluted fish from a farm pond.

Chapter 3

LAKESIDE AND SEASIDE
MAY NOT BE ENOUGH

CASIMIR M. NIKEL

IF the chemically susceptible person must seek an aquatic environment, certain hazards associated with such a move should not be overlooked. The shoreline flora tends to produce abundant spore growth that often is harmful. Stagnant backwaters often breed algae, numerous microbial organisms, and spontaneous gas fumes. Such contaminants might be harmful to the chemically susceptible individual, especially when these contaminants become airborne and if they invade the hypersensitive person's domiciliary environment. Consequently, the body of water should be preferably surrounded by steep banks of rocky material with no bayous or potholes surrounding it.

The following case history illustrates how easily an uninformed decision can lead a chemically susceptible person into trouble:

CASE HISTORY 1. Mr. M decided to take a vacation on the seacoast in order to benefit from the fresh air associated with sea breezes. His first stop was at Cape Cod, Massachusetts. Making the Village of Sandwich his base of operations, he spent a pleasant week visiting historic spots in the area. No discomforting symptoms were observed, although Mr. M had known sensitivities to dusts and molds.

The following ten days were spent touring along the seacoast southward. Upon reaching the southern tip of New Jersey, Mr. M experienced profuse drainage from the eyes and nostrils. At Cape May he slept only two hours during the entire night. Mr. M also felt a general neuralgic misery that persisted unrelentingly, except for about an hour while crossing the Delaware Bay on a ferry.

Several differences in the environmental conditions seemed

not to coincide with the conditions experienced by Mr. M in the Cape Cod area. The following seemed to prevail: The temperatures were higher in the Delaware Bay area; the shoreline was full of inland stagnant bayous and ponds. Probably the other influence was due to the winds blowing off the land toward the ocean. The syndrome of allergenic symptoms continued until M's trip reached a point of about 100 miles inland on a westerly course from Virginia Beach, Virginia.

A review of Mr. M's experience pointed up one important factor. Proximity of a large body of water does not assure freedom from discomforting incitants for the chemically susceptible person. Environmental conditions are extremely variable. These variables might frustrate the hope for relief from discomfort despite the presumed best of circumstances.

It cannot be overemphasized that any move to a new location should be taken with extreme caution. In contemplation of a relocation of residence, a chemically susceptible person would find it advisable to avail himself of the services from an *environmental consultant* before deciding upon the new location. Such a technologist is acquainted with geographical elements related to health ecology.

Generally, an environmental consultant is qualified by training as well as by personal experience. He is capable of diagnosing the indoor environment as well as the geographical conditions surrounding it. He may, therefore, be unusually helpful in selecting a house in the new location if an existing domicile is intended at the new location, rather than building a new house. However, if new construction is intended, it is recommended that the environmental consultant review the plans, specifications, design, and structural materials to be used in the construction of the new house. This may be the ounce of prevention that will prevent a pound of costly remodeling immediately upon moving into the new home.

The following case history is presented to illustrate the magnitude of difficulty in choosing a compatible geographical location for the chemically susceptible individual:

CASE HISTORY 2. Mr. G lived in a metropolitan city, which will be referred to hereafter as Brus. This city had a population of 1 million persons. The climate of Brus was mild. The topography was an undulating region with a huge lake bordering the city on the north. The shoreline extended in excess of 100 miles eastward and a similar distance to the west. The width of the lake from south to north was in excess of 30 miles.

The area surrounding the city was a beautiful pastoral countryside. The nearest city eastward was 20 miles away. It had a population of fifteen thousand persons. To the south the farming area extended 40 miles to a city of one hundred thousand population. Westward, the rural area was sprinkled with small hamlets for 100 miles with one exception. Beginning at the western edge of Brus the shoreline of the lake slanted northwesterly, and at a location 30 miles distant, an industrial community was situated at the mouth of a river that emptied into the lake.

Mr. G moved to the city of Brus in the middle 1940s at the age of thirty-four. Although he had some undefined gastric discomforts, he was not considered as an allergenically sensitive person at that time. He was given a thorough medical examination prior to moving to Brus that indicated that Mr. G was in excellent health with the exception of some gastric enzyme deficiency. Acidulin® was prescribed and Mr. G was released to roam freely in the presumably healthful environment of Brus.

Mr. G's first house was 10 miles east of the center of the city of Brus. The prevailing winds in that region were from the west in the summer and from the northwest in the winter. Although the neighborhood in which Mr. G located was on the eastern edge of a 600-acre park it was obvious to Mr. G that the air was cleaner in the western half of the city than in the eastern half. This was due to several major steel mills and chemical factories located in a gorgelike valley that traversed Brus through its center from south to north. In view of these circumstances, Mr. G moved to the western half of the community in 1951.

In terms of what is considered conducive treatment for chemically susceptible patients, G's move was desirable. He was not suspected of allergic tendencies at this time. He was employed in a hospital as an executive; therefore, frequent medical progress checkups were availed. During the first six years in Brus, rheumatoid arthritis set in for Mr. G; therefore, he utilized various laboratory and radiology testing to pinpoint the cause of his problem. Nothing definitive was determined by these techniques.

At the new location of Brus in the western half of the city, Mr. G experienced progressively declining health. In 1957 he was diagnosed to be sensitive to house dust by the skin-scratch tests. Occasionally he experienced coughing seizures and a burning sensation in the chest due to fumes issuing from a nearby fertilizer manufacturing plant (2 miles distant). In 1965 Mr. G decided to move to what he considered a clean suburb. This was on the windward, westerly side of the area, 10 miles west of his location in the western half of Brus. Again this move should have been a recommended one for a chemically susceptible person, although Mr. G was not suspected of such a tendency at this time.

The suburb to which Mr. G moved was a totally residential community. It was surrounded by open farmland. The population was twenty-five thousand persons. The nearest industrial community was 25 miles northwest of this suburb. In view of the prevailing westerly winds, this should have been a reasonably acceptable location. However, Mr. G's health continued to decline.

Within three years following the move to the suburb, national awareness of general air pollution resulted in county-wide monitoring in the county of G's residence. This established a surprising situation. The suburb was determined to be experiencing the highest airborne particulate pollution in the entire county. This, of course, was contrary to all expectations under the circumstances described in this case history.

The explanation of air pollution in the suburb might have included several factors. It is likely that westerly winds fed a pall of soil and vegetation particulates from the farmland. Although it was never proven to be the contributing cause, the industrial community of thirty thousand population 25 miles to the northwest and several medium-sized factories in the intervening distance might also have contributed substantially to the high concentration of airborne particulates. Probably the major cause of the condition was due to excessive housing construction experienced in the suburb. It was undergoing an explosive growth. Despite its restriction barring air-polluting factories within its borders, its endemic activity of earth moving for housing construction was presumably producing unsuspected major air pollution.

Mr. G's health continued to deteriorate progressively under the circumstances described, and in 1972 he moved to another state for health reasons. Shortly thereafter, Mr. G was diagnosed to be chemically susceptible. Mr. G's inhalant sensitivity was put under control through specific ambient-chemical-extracting air depollution techniques. Following this, he experienced important health improvement very shortly in his new environment, which was supplemented with the chemically cleaned air.

The following conclusions can be drawn from this case history:

1. Based on the generally accepted principles for geographical selection of residency by a chemically susceptible person, Mr. G presumably made the correct moves.
2. Despite these moves Mr. G's health was not improved noticeably.
3. Subsequent developments indicated that Mr. G was not avoiding air pollution despite his seemingly appropriate relocations.
4. Mr. G seemingly lacked information about two important factors in his geographical evaluations —
   A. He did not know that he was sensitive to gaseous chemicals as well as to foods and to airborne particulates.
   B. He did not know the types of pollutants, nor the degree of their concentration, in the atmosphere of the geographical areas to which he was relocating.
5. Consequent to the foregoing, Mr. G's efforts for self-improvement proved to be fruitless.

Mr. G might have taken the following effective precautions:

1. Mr. G should have availed himself of the services of an ecologic clinician. Such a physician knows how to test for inhalant gaseous sensitivity, as well as how to test for particulate inhalants and for ingestive incitants. Having established gaseous sensitivity, Mr. G could have avoided

the pollutants of this nature.

2. Mr. G might also have utilized the services of an environmental consultant. Such a person is trained in determining types and concentrations of pollutants by air samplings. Such technologists are scarce, to be sure. Mr. G could have availed himself, however, of information from the county health department, since he lived in a community with such resources.

The difficulty experienced by Mr. G should not be interpreted to mean that the geographical approach to resolving the health problems of a chemically susceptible person is hopeless. It does suggest that moving about blindly is sometimes frustrating. Moving to the seashore or to a dry climate, for example, has been practiced for centuries by health seekers. The abundance of favorable results has produced ample evidence that geographical factors can be lifesaving. In the instance of chemical susceptibility, it is very important that the patient follow carefully the guidance of an *ecologic clinician.*

In the case of chemical susceptibility, it is very important to accomplish maximum avoidance by the victim of specific environmental pollutants. It is particularly true in the case of a patient sensitive to gaseous pollutants in the general and domiciliary air. One authority suggests that it would be a lesser drain on the total national resources to isolate chemically susceptible persons than to clean up adequately the city air pollution for such persons. This, of course, makes consideration of geographical relocation imperative. From the experience of the people in the two case histories in this chapter, it appears that proximity of a lake or any major body of water is no assurance of an ecologically healthful environment.

Chapter 4

SITE SELECTION
AND THE FOUNDATION

Casimir M. Nikel

IN a previous chapter Doctor MacLennan discussed the geographical factors for situating the ecological, healthful house. In view of the generally publicized air pollution hazards, the reasons for such a discussion are obvious. To be concerned, however, with the foundation may seem less obvious, yet the hazards that involve the ecology of the foundation and the ecology of the construction site can be equally harmful.

Regarding the topic of health ecology, it is important to recognize that the environment is microscopic as well as macroscopic. That the environment is not a simple entity is becoming increasingly evident. The environment is not only the world surrounding us — it is also a world inside of us.

The biological cell is a good example of the microscopic internal environment. A single cell, like the mitochondrion floating in the protoplasm, possesses a universe of its own. Inside its outer shell is a veritable laboratory of enzymes. This tiny microscopic cell has an environment distinctive to itself. As long as this environment is not invaded by a harmful chemical, the respiration of the cell remains intact. If this mitochondrion is invaded by a fraction of urethane, it has been observed to cause a mutation resulting in a cancerous growth (1).

The illustration of the mitochondrion suggests a spectrum of environments. In fact, the macroscopic ecosphere is split up by the environmentalists into such separate entities as the atmosphere, biosphere, hydrosphere, etc. Close examination, of course, reveals a range of environments with which every living being must contend. The ecologic spectrum of the chemically susceptible person's house environment is even more complex than is normally suspected.

The house environment is extremely complex. It is affected by many influences. For example, the sun rays coming through the window can release an odorless gas into the house from chemically unstable draperies. On the other hand, the body heat of a person sitting on the polyfoam rubberoid upholstery of a sofa can also release harmful gas and surround the person. A common source of harmful pollution originates with heating systems, wall paints, adhesives used in fabrication of furniture, and adhesives used for installation of floor tiles and similar fixtures. Many forms of pollution from living activities and from emanations of physical objects within the house itself modify the house environment.

For practical purposes the discussion in Chapter 2 was separated from the discussion in this chapter. That discussion dealt with the regional environment as well as with the immediate neighborhood environment. In this chapter the emphasis will be on ecologic factors in choosing the house site and the foundation. Although the lot and the foundation are on the outside of the building, their influence can affect the inside environment of the house. This will become increasingly evident as the discussion in this chapter progresses.

Often quite common pollutants are overlooked in the house environment. This is partly true because the disturbing symptoms appear a long time after exposure to the pollution has occurred (2). Also, some of the pollution is invisible, such as nonodorous fumes. If an individual, however, exercises continual vigilance with the aid of his physician, most of the harmful pollutants can be identified. Once identification has been established, a proper course for correction can be developed. It cannot be overemphasized that perpetual alertness to environmental factors is a must.

A case history made available recently illustrates how important perpetual alertness is in order to cope successfully with ecological health problems. This particular case history, interestingly, relates to the house-foundation factor. It is presented here to underscore the point for perpetual alertness: Mr. R's modern suburban home was built with termite shields flush with the outside of the wall, instead of sticking out at least 2 inches. Earth was filled around the house on one side to a depth of 1 foot above the termite shield. It should have been kept at least 8 inches below the shield. Consequently, a limited infestation of termites entered the house at one point.*

> To combat the infestation the home owner put some chlordane outside the block foundation to kill the termites. Sufficient fumes from the chlordane seeped through the foundation to precipitate a reaction in a chemically sensitive member of the family. When this was added to the numerous other chemical exposures in the home, such as bushels of cans and bottles containing various chemicals, wall-to-wall carpet with underlayment, wall paper paste, fungicide, etc., the patient's tolerance for offensive chemicals was overwhelmed.
>
> Unless installed properly, termite shields do not work. Proper installation can be quite demanding, especially around stairs and entry ways. It is better to have the inconvenience of taking the step or two up into the house, which the proper installation of a termite shield requires, than to have the inconvenience of termites or having a house that people cannot live in because of the need to use pesticides. Ordinarily the mechanical method of termite prevention is preferred over the chemical method even in a family with no established chemical sensitivity.

The foregoing case history indicates only one element of the foundation for an ecologically healthful house. Other elements will be presented in this chapter. It cannot be overemphasized, however, that no detail is too small or too insignificant in the construction of an ecologically healthful house. And above all, the immediate construction site, as well as the type of foundation, bears intense scrutiny before the first shovel of earth is turned or the final decision is made to purchase the proposed lot for the house.

CONSIDERATIONS IN THE CONSTRUCTION SITE SELECTION

Patients who receive treatment for *hypersensitivity* from competent physicians hear repeatedly that avoidance of *incitants* is

---

*Used by permission from Francis Silver. Part of lecture presented to the 9th Seminar of The Society for Clinical Ecology.

preferred over the treatment of symptoms. Some incitants are impossible to avoid. Pollens are present everywhere, for example. The only way to avoid them totally is to live in a glass jar that is supplied with absolutely clean air. This, of course, is impractical.

For the long term benefit of the patient, the question arises as to what should be avoided in regard to the construction site and the foundation. In response to this question, it is necessary to determine what might be the incitant potential at the proposed construction site. Generally there are four types of incitants. Classed by the manner of exposure, the incitants are the following: contactants, ingesta, injectibles, and inhalants.

The contactants and the inhalants obviously are the most likely offenders on a house lot. Precautions should be taken, therefore, to select a site with a minimum of contactant and inhalant incitants on the construction site. Sites free of all incitants may not be feasible. If this is the case, the patient's physician should be consulted to determine which pollutants can be tolerated on the site after it is fully landscaped. These are some classes of incitants:

1. Forest droppings	6. Molds
2. Grasses and weeds	7. Rodents
3. Ground fumes	8. Soil
4. Insects and vermin	9. Trees
5. Landfills	10. Water

Some of these sources of pollution may have area-wide involvement. If they had not been spotted in the geographical survey, they still might be present on the actual proposed construction site. Ground fumes, for example, might be present from leaky gas lines on adjacent lots or from the street-line gas pipes. One city to which this author travels frequently is reported to use hydrogen sulfide to odorize the utility gas. This, over a prolonged period, has resulted in corrosive damage, presumably to the underground gas pipes. The over-all effect has created a ground-fume situation that is intolerable to hypersensitive persons in that particular city. A prominent and competent ecologic physician in this city is desperately urging many of his patients to move out of that city. He himself has built a house approximately 20 miles away from the city in order to escape the ground-fume problem. His office is equipped with air de-pollution units in all exam and treatment rooms. He is spending hours of his valuable time monitoring pollution, servicing depollution machinery, and trying to convince his patients that there is legitimately such a problem as harmful ground-fume pollution in their beloved city.

Some individuals who do not suffer from chemical suscepti-bility may take the foregoing lightly. They might say, "Such things are rare and probably impossible." On the other hand, there are other sources of ground-fume pollution. Conse-quently surveying for potential troublesome pollution on a proposed house construction site should not be done carelessly.

To clarify the potential hazards of the hypersensitive indi-vidual the ten sources listed earlier will be briefed individually.

Forest Droppings

Forest droppings frequently are loaded with numerous inci-tants. Such droppings may contain an accumulated mat several inches thick of nature's waste. This mat consists mostly of leaves and dead branches. It is richly endowed with molds. The forest mat has served as a cemetery for dying birds, rodents, insects, snakes, and other wildlife. This conglomerate of dead flora and dead fauna is a lethal source of trouble for the hyper-sensitive person. During the wet season the deep mat of forest droppings spawns various molds. During the dry season the mat becomes a source of powdered incitants that are ready for airborne aggravation to the hypersensitive individual.

In highly populated areas forest mats and droppings have been stripped to the topsoil, therefore, hazards of this type are minimal. Chemically sensitive persons, however, often move into rural areas to escape industrial pollution. They are un-aware of the hazards of these thick forest mats. Such fugitives from the city may clear a house construction site and landscape it beautifully, but overlook the hundreds of acres surrounding their house site with a literal dumping ground of nature. Forest droppings, therefore, should be given serious consideration in any survey for the proposed ecologically healthful house site.

Grasses and Weeds

Grasses and weeds are not only a direct source of incitants for the hypersensitive person, but they are also indicators of other factors that might cause trouble. For example, the presence of cattails and sawgrass suggests swampy conditions. The soggy condition of an extinct swamp might contribute a perpetual dose of slime molds. Filling in such low spots with clean soil will not necessarily eliminate the probable mold growth from the subsurface reserve.

Of the 4,500 species of grasses identified throughout the world, 1500 of them grow in the United States (3). Hansel indicates that only a small number of them are serious troublemakers for the so-called hay fever sufferer. Unfortunately those grasses which are offenders consist mostly of agriculturally grown grains. Wheat smut, for instance, and wheat pollen contribute heavily to the problem of the hypersensitive patient in widely spread areas of the United States. Confining the survey to the construction site, the weed problem, however, is generally the more serious incitant for the hypersensitive individual.

Weeds are self-cultivated, consequently they predominate on a proposed house site. If the site is located in an undeveloped area, such weeds are valuable as indicators of the predominant weeds indigenous to the region. Although such weeds can be removed from the site by the process of stripping, it does not assure that the future hypersensitive home owner will escape the harmful airborne contaminants of weeds in the surrounding area.

Identifying the weeds on the proposed site is important. If done correctly, it can assist in determining the environmental compatability of the future house for the hypersensitive person. Your physician can test you for your tolerance to the particular weeds on your proposed house site. If you are not sensitive to them, that is a most encouraging determination. It assures you not only of your immediate location, but it also suggests that the weeds of the region are not likely to bother you.

Ground Fumes

Ground fumes have been discussed to some extent in a previous paragraph. It must be noted, however, that fumes are not confined to utility gas only. Nearby oil fields, oil refineries, sewerage plants, cesspools, and incinerators are troublesome fume sources. Leaf burners are common troublemakers, especially if they are used for trash burning also. Always assure yourself that a neighbor is not operating an open-type waste-burning unit.

Swamp gas suggests nature-produced fumes, which can be harmful to the hypersensitive person. Sometimes a natural gas area may not be commercially viable, but it may be seeping fumes into the atmosphere and thereby creating a harmful condition for the hypersensitive person. Such conditions should be avoided. In fact, it may be of benefit to do so for those who are not identified as hypersensitive. Increasingly, it appears that continued exposure over a prolonged time develops sensitivity in individuals who formerly have not been chemically sensitive.

In line with this concept of ground fumes, a group of physicians recently surveyed indicated that the safe distance from a gas well for the hypersensitive person is 10 to 50 miles. The distance probably depends to a large degree on the number of gas wells in a given field. The degree of sensitivity also might contribute to the distance a person should live from a gas well. Nevertheless, it is definite that the house must be located upstream of the prevailing winds for maximum safety to the hypersensitive person. In evaluating a proposed house site, be sure that it is free of ground fumes.

Insects and Vermin

Insects and vermin are more troublesome than is commonly suspected. This is due to the difficulty of identifying the source of symptoms, except in the visible stinging and biting types of insects. Mueller reports that despite a 4,000 year history of death due to insect bites, patients suffering life-threatening reactions from insect bites "are still considered to be in the category of medical curiosities" (4).

Vermin pollutants can be classified in various ways. For convenience of the hypersensitive person, they can be classed the following ways: (1) inhalant and contact types, and (2) stinging and biting types. The latter of these is most easily traced to the hypersensitive person's reaction. The former is so seldom visible that it is almost impossible to discover as an incitant. For example, Mueller reports an interesting observation about inhalant reactions related to insects, as presented by S. M. Feinberg, et al. (4). He states that "inhalation or contact by sensitive persons with microscopic bits of insects may cause; asthma, rhinitis, conjunctivitis or atopic dermatitis." Brown also relates an interesting case history along this line of inhalant and contact sensitivity to insects (5). He tells of one situation in which rat mites invaded the house by traveling from the basement along the plumbing and electrical pipe runs and thereby created a harmful infestation for the patient. This resulted in serious illness.

Based on findings by responsible scientists and physicians, it seems imperative that the foundation site for an ecologically healthful house must be given a careful examination for various insects, mites, chiggers, worms, termites, and vermin known to be inimical to the patient's health (6).

Another observation seems in order at this point. Insects and vermin are doubly troublesome to hypersensitive persons. Firstly, direct contact can be fatal. Secondly, the pesticides used to rid the premises of vermin can be devastating to the hypersensitive person. The case history from Silver (which was referred to earlier in this chapter) illustrates the latter point quite dramatically.

Based on personal experience, it seems that few patients have the capability to adequately evaluate the proposed house site. It is advisable, therefore, for the hypersensitive person to utilize the services of an *environmental consultant* before making the final decision on a house site. If soil borings are needed, such a specialist has the expertise for it. Foundation sites that appear to possess historic subsurface forest droppings may merit soil boring samples. This would verify whether concentrated deposits of vermin are present. By this means, one might prevent building on a site that would produce unanticipated vermin infestation after completion of construction.

Landfills

Landfills are becoming a more serious problem, especially in metropolitan areas where housing land developments become larger and housing land sites are becoming increasingly scarce. Small depressions on a single lot can be filled with clean soil from a known source. This kind of landfill would pose no problem. Increasingly in metropolitan communities, landfills include trash and sometimes garbage. Such waste materials are used to fill in major cavernous areas and lowlands. This type of landfill poses serious problems. It attracts rodents and insects and breeds molds. Discussion of such elements in other parts of this commentary would suggest that any construction site with landfill should be avoided. Even after the visible presence of rodents, insects, and molds has been ruled out, the residual pollution of such things as dander, carcass particles, and dehydrated spores may remain on a landfill site. Spontaneous gas pollution from decaying landfill is also a problem for the chemically susceptible individuals. Therefore, landfill locations remain potential hazards for the hypersensitive person and should be avoided by any means.

Molds

Molds are probably the most common troublemakers for the hypersensitive person, generally because of their widespread presence. Doctor Hansel's discussion of molds relates them to trees, grasses, weeds, dusts, and foods (7). Problems with food often result from additives, such as yeast in breads, pastries, beer, and soft drink beverages like root beer. Frequently, molds in foods and drinks arise spontaneously. Especially is this true of fruits that ferment easily. What appears to be spontaneous development of molds is also commonly found in settled dusts and in building structures.

The growth of molds is not fully understood. It is commonly assumed that high humidity causes mold growth. This does not seem to be completely true according to a national survey performed by the Research Council of the American Academy of Allergy. Quoting from that report, Hansel indicates that certain specific species of molds are several hundred percent more abundant in Albuquerque, New Mexico than in Miami, Florida (8). Considering that Albuquerque is in an arid climate and that Miami is on the seacoast with massive offshore swampy areas, the reverse incidence of molds should be expected.

Local experience in the arid areas indicates that molds tend to grow best when the temperatures are cool and the area is shielded from direct sunlight exposure. In New Mexico the temperatures drop twenty to thirty degrees each night, which provides the favorable environment for mold growth. In Florida the night temperatures remain high; consequently, molds are sparse despite humid conditions there.

Now the question may be raised, "How does this relate to house foundations and hypersensitive persons?" Simply, it suggests that the construction of an ecologically healthful house must avoid conditions conducive to molds associated with foundation structures. Certain conditions on the proposed site must be avoided. Displacement of water deposits with landfill may create a permanent source of mold pollution. A layer of clay or sand may cover over a soggy subsurface that can become an incubator for molds.

The coeditors of this book performed a survey of the physicians holding membership in the Society for Clinical Ecology. Seventy-five percent of the respondents indicated that soggy soil at the construction site should be avoided. This may have been also partly the reason why 50 percent of the same respondents preferred hilltop locations for the home of a chemically susceptible person. Such professional opinion should be ample warning to avoid poorly drained construction sites, which might breed molds harmful to hypersensitive persons. It should be also noted that mold growth is characteristic of certain types of house foundations, despite reasonably dry construction sites; therefore, it is very important to prevent mold pollutants from the house foundation source. The technology of constructing proper house foundations will be discussed later in this chapter.

Rodents

At first thought, rodents, as a source of pollution for the hypersensitive, may seem unimportant and easily controlled. One might think mice and rats are a source of physical pollution; however, they may be one of the undiscovered, more complex sources of pollution that results in numerous cases of chronic illness. This is primarily true because rodents are a more common source of infestation than is suggested by mice and rats only. This source of pollution is more important than cursory attention suggests. The most common rodents that might infest the environment for a hypersensitive person are chipmunks, gophers, rabbits, squirrels, and woodchucks, as well as the more commonly thought of mice and rats. Also, rodent infestation may seem unimportant for the hypersensitive because rodents have been associated principally with contagious diseases. Such contagions have been identified with plague, tetanus, typhus, etc. Diseases from such contagions have been, of course, reasonably controlled.

In actuality the hypersensitive person may suffer from remote contact to rodents and not from direct contact, as is generally true of contagion from rodents. Such remote contact is airborne. Individuals susceptible to reaction from animal dander conceivably may be inhaling dander produced by rodents in the neighborhood and may be unaware that it is causing their illnesses. This mechanism of airborne animal dander has been established in southwestern areas, where patients sensitive to cattle dander will suffer from this pollution despite separation from ranch locations by several miles distance.

To be sure, rodent pollution needs more research to be given important value in the hypersensitivity process. Identification of harmful reactions to rodents in the case of pets, however, suggests that more research of rodent pollution is advisable. Doctor Rapp lists mice, gerbils, rabbits, hamsters, and cats as a source of trouble for the hypersensitive person (9). The author of this chapter has known persons who were sensitive to house cats, and they were proven to be equally sensitive to wild cats.

This kind of clinical observation suggests the importance of rodent pollution. Probably the most important evidence in support of taking rodent pollution seriously at the house site of the hypersensitive is supported by some research recently reported in the *Annual Review of Allergy — 1972*. It is stated that "the inhalation of animal danders is one of the allergens involved in causing attacks of asthma" (10). What is true of urban children can be assumed as also likely of rural children who might be exposed to field rodents. It would seem to this author very important that rodent pollution be given consideration in the selection of a house site for the hypersensitive person.

Soil

Soil has not been generally incriminated by the classic allergists. Enough has been learned, however, about dust-related illness to make soil highly suspect in relation to site selection for the chemically hypersensitive person. Recently released information about *pneumoconioses* has cast enough light on the health problem with soil dusts that the federal government is now making an intensive study of the subject (12). About two dozen dusts, including farm soil, are known to be harmful to human health (13). Probably the most convincing argument for considering soil as a harmful pollutant to the hypersensitive person is the theory propounded by the late J. R. Howe, D.V.M. (14). He stated that we "hear talk of air, water and soil pollution. People tend to isolate these, but there is a great deal of interlinking with the soil." He illustrates the interlinkage by pointing out that ions in the drinking water become incorporated with bone and tissue structure of people and animals. Upon death, the ions of drinking water that became part of the body chemistry revert to the earth and intermingle with surface soil. Doctor Howe further emphasizes that "we must not think of air pollution as an entirely separate problem. Soil and water are vital factors in air pollution." When the soil has been impregnated by water with various chemicals, it has become a lethal factor in the environment of the hypersensitive person (15). Any such soil, when dry and airborne, can become intolerable to the hypersensitive individual. From this it is obvious that soil consideration is an important element in site selection.

Since information about soil incrimination is scanty, only elemental suggestions can be offered. The site for the home of a hypersensitive person should be surrounded by well-anchored soil. This may be effected by soil structure or by adequate sod covering. The soil should be of homogenous content, such as clay, uniform sand, or rocklike structure. This suggestion implies easier testing for sensitivity by the ecologic physician, if it is deemed necessary to assure maximum safety. Alluvial soil and aggregate soil should be avoided, since it would be more difficult to determine which portion of their contents caused trouble for the hypersensitive person.

Other approaches can be suggested to assure optimum safety regarding the soil in site selection. Number one is to locate in temporary quarters in the area of the contemplated site and reside there at least one year. The reason for suggesting a one year residence is due to windy seasons in some areas. During such periods the hypersensitive person will experience maximum exposure to airborne soil. Such exposure will tend to reveal any problems with sensitivity to soil in the area of the planned location. The second approach is to test the water from a shallow well in the area. Such a well tends to accumulate chemicals by leaching them from the surrounding soil. If the hypersensitive person should be susceptible to some of the chemicals in the surrounding soil, he is apt to react to those chemicals in the well water. It must be recognized, however, that this is only an approximate method of testing. Often a compound chemical in the soil, which in its dry state might be harmful, conceivably could become dissociated in the test water and lose its harmful effect. On the other hand, the converse effect may develop; therefore, exposure to shallow-well water is not completely certain. Nevertheless, it is not useless. In the total site evaluation, it is another way of trying to achieve hopefully satisfactory conditions. Although soil determination by this means is approximate, it is a sure way of determining that the available water will be compatible, even if later exposure to wind-driven soil proves it to be otherwise.

Trees

The love affair with trees that is exhibited by professional landscapers and the enthusiastic willingness of the potential home owner to join them suggest that the following discussion may be dangerous. Trees, nevertheless, have been incriminated as inimical to the chemically hypersensitive person. This is especially true of decorative trees. The following species of trees have been listed by various researchers as having wide-ranging effects on the hypersensitive: alder, ash, birch, cedar, elm, fir, hickory, maple, oak, pine, poplar, sycamore, and walnut (16).

The mechanism of pollution by trees is complex. It involves contactants and inhalants. Trees produce pollen, molds, fumes, and oily sap. All of these tree-originated substances, except the oily sap, may possibly become airborne. Hypersensitive persons inhaling pollens, tree-spawned molds, and tree-emanated fumes may experience chronic as well as acute distressing symptoms. Yet these victims are too often unable to trace their health problems to the pollution from trees.

Fumes from trees generally involve the *terpenes*. Most conifers produce such fumes. Socially, we have been conditioned to believe that the odors of cedar are sanitizing and healthful. In the survey that was mentioned earlier in this chapter one physician reported that cedar was the most harmful of all the conifers to his patients.

The survey we made requested the expression of preference for fifteen species of tree-grown wood. Interestingly 85 percent of the responding physicians approved the hardwoods, only 1.5 percent preferred softwoods, and 1 percent favored redwood in the resin species grouping. Thirty percent of the respondents expressed a definite rejection of resin woods within the environment of their patients. This is significant in view of the fact that the group surveyed consists of ecologic specialists in the treatment of various forms of allergy and chemical susceptibility. Clinical experience indicates that hypersensitive persons should avoid conifer trees and wood products derived from them, unless tolerance for such exposure has been established by a physician as well as by personal contact through repeated exposure and careful observation.

The most common illness reported from tree pollution is asthma. Skin diseases are also a common reaction, especially in the case of poison oak. One physician reported a possibility of renal disease as correlative to an infection from poison oak.

There is a brighter side to the subject of tree pollution, however. One authority indicated that flowering trees (fruit-bearing variety, for example) do not depend on airborne pollenization (17). This should produce relief from tree pollens. Chestnut, locust, and willow also were reported to be free of pollen pollution. Then too, chemical hypersensitivity is not general in many cases. A person may have his physician test him for sensitivity to some hardwood decorative trees to determine his tolerance for them. This group includes ash, hickory, mahogany, oak, rock maple, and walnut. The second-best grouping consists of softwoods, which include birch, cherry, poplar, and sugar maple. Norway maple is also frequently tolerable. If a home owner is anxious to landscape the site for his house with trees, it would be advisable for him to be tested for the specific specie of trees he has chosen before investing in a planting that will prove later to be harmful to his health.

Water

The question of water will be discussed comprehensively later in this book, therefore, this author shall not review it in depth. Also the problem of water-logged house sites has been mentioned earlier in the discussion of molds. However, water spawns other pollution than molds. Vegetation submerged in water often produces hydrocarbon gases, which can float into the domestic area of a hypersensitive person. Such nearby conditions in ponds, creeks, and marshes must be avoided. Another form of inimical pollution for the hypersensitive person is water-spawned insects. Despite the fact that human life cannot survive without water, it is nevertheless important to consider water pollution in the selection of a house site.

Other factors besides pollution from the ten sources discussed heretofore are equally important in the home site selection. Such factors involve socioeconomic elements. The do-it-yourselfer should be alert to such factors as building codes, zoning requirements, deed restrictions, etc. *Your Dream Home — How to Build it for Less* is an excellent resource for the do-it-yourselfer regarding socioeconomic factors in site selection (18). It seems to me, however, that a home-owner builder should not depend exclusively on information listed heretofore, nor on information gleaned from other books. Consultation with the following specialists seems advisable: physician, *house-call consultant,* architect, banker or other financing agency representative, and a competent attorney who specializes in real estate contracts and tax laws.

THE ELEMENTS OF THE FOUNDATION

After the house site has been chosen and purchased, the hypersensitive person is faced with numerous construction details, even if he contracts the construction of the proposed house. Such detail is greatly different than that of conventional house construction. The difference is in the limitation of the purpose for a conventional house, which is basically built for thermal comfort.

The house for the hypersensitive person must provide ecologic healthfulness in addition to thermal comfort. This is a new dimension. Ecologic healthfulness requires avoidance from ambient pollution. Optimum avoidance is only possible if ambient pollution has been prevented during the construction process.

Awareness of how important prevention of ambient pollution is probably poses the greatest problem in construction of a house for the hypersensitive person. Although the prospective home owner of such a house may possess adequate awareness, the architects, contractors, material suppliers, and other persons involved in house construction generally are unaware that the slightest deviation can defeat the ultimate achievement of ecologic healthfulness. It would probably be advisable to provide the architect and the general contractor with information about the effect of indoor invisible smog before planning and construction is started (19). Supplementing such orientation with supervision by an ecologic clinician and house-call consultant might assure the achievement of optimum ecologic healthfulness in the proposed house.

The first construction component one faces in building an ecologically healthful house is the foundation. The following discussion shall include the floor and footers in the general term of foundation. There are predominantly three types of foundations utilized for house construction in our country:

1. Pier- and post-type
2. Basement-type
3. Concrete slab-type

For the hypersensitive person, an important item to avoid in foundation structures is mold growth. The first two foundation types listed above are most susceptible to spawning harmful molds. The concrete slab foundation is the reverse. It is suited for developing conditions that will minimize transfer of molds into the living area. Consequently, the following discussion will deal principally with the concrete slab-type of foundation, although many important factors must be considered in the selection of a house foundation. Narrow and short house lots, for example, press for utilization of basement structures. Dry climates and arid, dry house sites might dictate a pier-and-post foundation, with some precautionary measures. But for most conditions and circumstances, the concrete slab foundation is preferred.

An ecologic factor often overlooked within the house is the breathing process of a house. There is a movement of air into the house, out of the house, and through the house by other pathways than the usual air-conditioning system, the heating system, windows, and doors. Backdrafts through planned vents and through structural fissures are common pathways for air infiltration into the house environment. The fireplace and exhaust vents in bathrooms are too frequently backdrafting pathways. Because of negative air pressure within the house, the outside, heavier atmosphere tries to force its way into the house by these various pathways (20). On a windy day, a test can be made of this by placing the back of the hand near the door latch or near an electrical outlet. This will indicate a jet of air blowing in through these crevicelike pathways. It is important to recognize that the air entering through the electrical outlet first had to pass through the wall space in order to travel through the electrical outlet. The intrawall space has stale dust and often molds in it, which pollute the passing air; therefore, through this house-breathing process the occupant within the house comes in contact unknowingly with serious incitants.

Linda Clark reports a case history that illustrates how the breathing process of a house can insidiously cause trouble for a hypersensitive person (21). The patient in this instance was afflicted with "small itching blisters on the palms of his hands." His physician diagnosed the problem as a sensitivity to molds. The patient insisted that there was no mold pollution in his house. The ailment was of ten years' duration when the patient decided to remodel the foundation of his house. After the house was elevated with jacks, it was discovered that there was a mold accumulation under the floor. Replacing the wood floor with a concrete slab resulted in elimination of the itching blisters.

From the foregoing example it is obvious that the breathing process of a house can cause a problem similar to the one Linda Clark reported. Consequently, the interacting forces of the outdoor environment with the indoor environment can create ecologic complexity as yet unsuspected.

We are reasonably sure that heat and air movement modify the ambient ecology of a house. For the hypersensitive person it is important, therefore, to consider every detail of the indoor environment and its interlocking relationship with every nook and cranny within the entire structure as well as the inter-locking relationship with the outdoor environment. With these thoughts in mind, we shall proceed to the discussion of the foundation factors in constructing an ecologically healthy house.

Probably the simplest foundation, in light of the foregoing, is a slab of concrete poured directly on the ground. It is an established fact of earth physics, however, that ground temperatures below the frost line remain about 55°F constantly. This is a favorable temperature for mold growth. Furthermore, the absence of sunlight under a foundation provides an ideal environment for mold growth. It is important, therefore, that special precautions be taken even in the case of the most preferred type of foundation.

To avoid, or at least to minimize, the possibility of mold growth under the house, a layer of gravel should be poured under the concrete slab. The thickness should be governed by the prevailing rainfall, the natural water table level, and the special conditions prevailing on the construction site. Gravel bed thickness may range from 4 inches to 20 inches according to the opinion survey mentioned earlier in this chapter. The latter thickness seems excessive, and if moisture levels are such that they suggest a one-foot deep gravel bed, then additional mechanical drainage seems needed.

Mechanical drainage can be effected in different ways. The most common system is a leach bed. Such a leach bed is constructed of a grid of perforated clay pipes. This grid is connected to a drain pipe. If the construction site is on a slope, gravity drainage will tend to dispose of the excess water to a lower-level area, hopefully one that is remote from the house. If the site is level and gravity drainage is not feasible, then a sump pit can be created at a lower level than the foundation (by digging a well for it), and the excess water will collect in the sump pit, at which point an electrically driven pump can take over to deliver the water to a street sewer or some other disposal point.

It should not be assumed that use of the mechanical drainage precludes the use of a gravel bed. For most efficient drainage, the perforated clay pipes of a leach bed should be covered by gravel. The gravel must be sufficiently coarse so that individual pebbles do not fall through the perforations into the clay pipes. The gravel bed should also fill in the spaces between the pipes, and spaced supports of concrete must be poured to keep the weight of the foundation slab from crushing the drain pipes.

When the entire leach bed of perforated pipe, gravel bed, and foundation supports has been completed, a layer of sand must be poured over this system. The sand is intended to protect a plastic sheeting, which must be laid over the entire foundation area. This plastic sheeting over the sand and under the foundation slab will serve as a vapor barrier. Such a system of isolating the concrete slab from the cool moisture beneath it will protect the porous concrete slab against becoming a mold supporting incubator.

Some physicians question the advisability of placing a plastic sheeting under the concrete slab. Their major concern is the emanating pollution from the plastic and the likelihood of this pollution working its way up through the porous concrete, as well as through the fissures that develop in the concrete slab upon settling. To the imperceptive person this seems to be an excessive concern. The author's personal experience, however, suggests that this is a legitimate possibility grounded in factual information. One thing is significant in this respect — chemically stable plastics are available. Experimentation with the emanating plastics for the moon trip spacecraft has established that some plastics are quite stable below the 70° thermal level (23). Consequently, the use of heavy plastic sheeting for a vapor barrier under the house foundation seems to pose a lesser threat than potential mold pollution from the house foundation for a hypersensitive person.

In the construction of a slab foundation, sometimes the height of the slab in relation to the surrounding soil is not given adequate attention. Home owners who prefer a basement-less house generally dislike steps. Too often, therefore, such houses are constructed on slabs so low that the bottom of the building wall is only a few inches above the groundfill. Occasionally, the wall structure actually touches the ground back-fill, which leaves the house extremely vulnerable to termite invasion. Treatment of such an invasion with chemical pesticides can be extremely harmful to the chemically susceptible person. The case history from Silver, which was quoted earlier in this chapter, is a prime example of why it is better to build the foundation slab with some steps above the surrounding groundfill. As has been mentioned earlier, a mechanical control of termites is preferred over chemical pesticides.

A more complex house foundation is a basement or a crawl space. Such a foundation has some important disadvantages that are not present in the slab-type foundation. Basements and crawl spaces provide a convenient storage space that too often becomes a trash-collecting dumping ground. A basement or crawl space full of junk becomes too difficult to clean. Neglected sanitation in basements and crawl spaces results in dust accumulation, which becomes a lethal source of incitants for the hypersensitive person.

The most serious handicap of the basement and crawl space cavity is its mold-breeding capacity. The temperatures in such ancillary spaces are generally low enough to sustain mold growth. The thermal differential from the occupied space above and from the ground temperatures below the basement is such that it generates indigenous humidity within the ancillary space underneath the house. The prevailing temperatures, especially at night, within a basement are suitable for mold growth. It would seem, therefore, that no unheated basement should be contemplated for a hypersensitive person. If such an ancillary space is overwhelmingly desired, the home owner should be prepared to maintain a 70° temperature all year around within the basement, unless no member of the family is susceptible to the effect of molds.

BIBLIOGRAPHY

1. Warburg, Otto: On the origin of cancer cells. *Science, 123* (2191):309-314, 1956.
2. Sherman, W.B., and Kessler, W.R.: *Allergy in Pediatric Practice.* St. Louis, Mosby, 1957, pp. 242-247.
   Hansel, French K.: *Clinical Allergy.* St. Louis, Mosby, p. 302.
3. Hansel, *Clinical Allergy,* p. 143.
4. Mueller, H.L.: *Symposium on Pediatric Allergy.* Philadelphia, Saunders, 1959, vol. 6, #3, pp. 917-918.
5. Brown, Halla: *Annual Review of Allergy — 1973.* Flushing, New York, Med Exam, p. 476.
6. Sherman and Kessler, *Allergy in Pediatric Practice,* 1957, pp. 53-60.
7. Hansel, *Clinical Allergy,* pp. 663-664.
8. Hansel, *Clinical Allergy,* p. 175.
9. Rapp, Doris J.: *Allergies & Your Child.* New York, HR&W, p. 223.
10. Frazier, Claude A. (Ed.): *Annual Review of Allergy — 1972.* Flushing, New York, Med Exam, p. 19.
11. Frazier, *Annual Review of Allergy — 1972,* pp. 24-25.
12. *Introduction to Lung Diseases,* 5th ed., 1973, pp. 87-98. Available from the American Lung Association.
13. Nikel, C.M.: *Breathing for Survival.* Hicksville, New York, Exposition, 1975, pp. 81-82.
14. *Archives for Clinical Ecology.* Society for Clinical Ecology, 1971, vol. 2, p. 22. Available from D.B. Warnock, Executive Secretary, 70 E. Meadow Lane, Edwardsville, Illinois 62025.
15. *Archives for Clinical Ecology,* p. 23.

16. Hill, L.W., and Mueller, H.L.: *Pediatr Clin North Am, 6* (3):844, August 1959.
17. Rapp, *Allergies & Your Child,* p. 6.
18. Cobb, Hubbard: *Your Dream Home: How to build it for less?,* Woodland Hills, California, Wise Pub, 1972, pp. 8-23.
19. Nikel, *Breathing for Survival,* p. 36.
20. Nikel, *Breathing for Survival,* pp. 109-110.
21. Clark, Linda: from summary of a Handbook on the Most Common Ailments. *Let's Live,* August 1973, p. 80.
22. Randolph, Theron G.: *Human Ecology and Susceptibility to the Chemical Environment,* 4th ed. Springfield, Thomas, 1972, p. 106.
23. Ball Brothers Research Corporation: Contamination ranking lists for materials, TR 70-10. *BBRC Study.* Boulder, Colorado, December 21, 1970. Available from Ball Brothers Research Corp.

Chapter 5

ECOLOGY OF THE SHELL STRUCTURE

CASIMIR M. NIKEL

THE following discussion will be limited to ecology only. Structure will be considered only in its relative effect upon the occupant's health.

As a structure, the shell of a house consists principally of three major components. They are doors, windows, and wall sections. Each of the components is related to the health of a hypersensitive individual. Each contributes in a different way, but all can contribute detrimentally to the quality of the air the hypersensitive person inhales.

The engineering structural factors will not be given technical consideration. Primarily the technicalities will be left out, because the shell structure is important to the engineer in terms of physical factors only. Generally, the engineer looks at the wall as a support for the ceiling, the windows, and the doors. Technically, the wall must have the strength to resist the stresses of swinging doors, the impact of the weather (the blasts of the wind and hail), while maintaining thermal comfort. The windows are expected to transmit light, and the doors to provide easy entrance and exit. In addition to the foregoing physical factors, the engineer and architect find esthetics important in the construction of the shell for a house, but they seldom face the responsibility of assuring a healthful impact on the occupants.

Normally, the engineer is concerned about the comfort of the occupants, but health considerations are merely a by-product of the engineers' endeavors. *Clinical ecology* specialists, on the other hand, are aware that a relationship to the health, especially for the hypersensitive individual, exists from the impacts associated with the shell structure of a house. The detrimental impacts are effected by two important phenomena — one is the process of *outgassing* by the materials utilized in the construction of the shell structure; the other is *structural respiration.* Both of these phenomena are recent discoveries and of much greater importance than one might suspect.

The terms *outgassing* and *structural respiration* require reasonably precise definition in order to maintain a clear understanding of the subsequent discussion. They will, therefore, be defined in the language of this author. Technical proof of the terms will be left to others. However, refinement of the meaning in the definition will have been made by competent professionals in the fields of science and medicine. The reader, therefore, may accept the terms with assurance of their reliability.

OUTGASSING. The process of slow and invisible disintegration of a physical material in molecular form and its diffusion into the surrounding air. The material might consist of synthetic fabric, paint, adhesive, floor tile, etc. The molecular portion of such a disintegrating material becomes airborne, and when it is inhaled by a hypersensitive person, the gaseous particles produce toxic reactions.

STRUCTURAL RESPIRATION. The exchange of air between the outside and the inside of the house through structural barriers intended to keep out the outside air. This unplanned atmospheric exchange produces toxic effects in the hypersensitive individual.

To portray the relationship of outgassing and structural-respiration and its effect upon the hypersensitive individual, each of the three major components of the shell structure will be reviewed separately.

WALL SECTION

The wall section of the shell structure contributes to problems of the hypersensitive individual through both of the previously defined phenomena. Outgassing is the principal culprit in this instance. This outgassing is mostly contributed by surface-treatment materials applied to inner walls. Because of the importance of this aspect of the shell-structure ecology, each of the wall-treatment materials will be reviewed individually.

Plaster

In applying-form, plaster is a pasty material made up of water and a caustic calcium oxide often mixed with magnesia. This pasty material is applied to the inner-wall surface with a trowel. When the applied portion is thoroughly seasoned by air-drying exposure, it becomes a chemically stable and hardened surface of exquisite whiteness. Most hypersensitive individuals can tolerate this kind of wall treatment.

For esthetic reasons the plastered inner walls are generally painted. Modern paints are mostly derived from petrochemicals and are highly volatile. This volatility results in an outgassing that disturbs most hypersensitive persons. Some of the paints outgas indefinitely. Such paints should be avoided completely. Some paints such as calcimines and acrylic paints seem to have a limited outgassing period. Following this outgassing, they may become tolerable to a hypersensitive individual. It is, however, not certain that all hypersensitive persons can tolerate calcimines and acrylic paints, therefore, a test in an isolated room should be performed before deciding on a specific paint brand for the entire project. Such a test should be performed in a facility available for the test, but one in which the hypersensitive individual is not committed to live indefinitely, should it become evident that the paint under test is intolerable.

Plasterboard

Plasterboard, a wall-veneering material, comes in panel form and is sometimes referred to as drywall or gypsum board. Plasterboard is composed principally of material similar to the lime substances of troweled plaster, which was discussed in a previous paragraph. However, in the plasterboard the lime substance is encased in a strong paper binding to form a panel approximately one-half inch in thickness.

Heretofore, plasterboard was considered to be safe for the hypersensitive individual. Recently, however, clinical ecologists have observed some disturbing effects. Investigation has not been conclusive, but the paper portion of the plasterboard has been incriminated. The latest findings suggest that the chemicals used for fireproofing the paper portion of the plasterboard causes outgassing.

A hypersensitive person should be advised to test himself for tolerance to a specific production lot of plasterboard before approving it for wall treatment in his home. Surveys suggest that not all factories use the same fireproofing chemicals. Therefore, a hypersensitive person might tolerate one chemical, but not another that is used in fabrication of plasterboard. Consequently, a pretesting might prevent a costly, but unacceptable investment. One physician found it necessary to seal in the offensive plasterboard, which was outgassing, with an overlay of ceramic tile in order to tolerate the atmosphere of his private office. This suggests how costly it may become when corrections are necessary due to unwarranted initial decisions.

It should be also noted that plasterboard requires decorating treatment. Its appearance is less attractive than troweled plaster. Consequently, the problem of paints and sheet-type decorating materials must be given additional consideration as an ecologic factor. Later discussion in this chapter will review some of the difficulties with decorating wall board.

Wallpaper

Wallpaper is less popular than during the earlier decades of this century. Despite its popularity during "Grandma's" era, wallpapering has its hazards also for the hypersensitive individual. Firstly, the printed decoration on the paper is made with outgassing types of inks and paints. These decorations, in addition to the adhesives required for the paper to stick to the wall, produce seriously harmful outgassing for the hypersensitive person. It should not be presumed that the outgassing can be locked in by the paper — the porosity of the paper is sufficient to allow passage of any molecular outgassing by pastes, glues, and other forms of adhesives.

Resorting to homemade adhesives is not a foolproof escape from the outgassing process. Some clinical ecologists report a mold growth associated with water-soluble pastes. Molds can be as troublesome as outgassing chemicals to the hypersensitive individual. Therefore, one might escape the outgassing hazard by use of homemade pastes, but if one is not resistant to molds an equal health hazard may be created.

Since the wallpapering process provides so many hazards, it seems that a hypersensitive person should approach this form of wall treatment with extreme caution.

Vinylsheeting

Plastic materials made of vinyl have been incriminated as disturbing to hypersensitive persons. It is not certain whether it is the vinyl itself or the *plasticizing* chemicals used to make the fabric pliable that are the causative chemicals in hypersensitive reactions. Sufficient clinical evidence exists to rule out vinylsheeting for wall treatment in the house of a hypersensitive person.

In addition to the basic stock material of vinylsheeting, the necessary adhesive to apply the sheeting to the wall is also a source of danger. Most of the adhesives used to apply the sheeting are of petrochemical derivation. This provides a high potential for outgassing.

It is suggested that a hypersensitive individual shun the use of vinylsheeting, unless he is absolutely sure from previous experience that a specific brand of the sheeting, and a specific stock lot of it, is tolerable. It is also worth noting that one should be certain of tolerating the specific brand and the specific stock lot of the adhesive to be used for a specific project.

Wood

Wood comes in two forms as wall-treatment material, i.e. as boards and as panels. Both may be in virgin stock, which will require painting or varnishing. On-site applied paints and varnishes outgas temporarily. Some paints may outgas indefinitely. Generally, varnish can be tolerated after a few weeks of seasoning. However, this method should not be accepted without reservation. Confirmation for tolerance to a specific product with pretesting by the hypersensitive individual is recommended.

The prefinished wood stock wall-veneers are sometimes preferred — especially the nonplywood panels, if the finish was kiln dried at high temperatures. The local lumberyards can provide specifications for particular prefinished brands of wood paneling. Additional consideration will elaborate on this aspect of the wall-structure treatment in Chapter 6 of this book. The foregoing has been presented principally to forewarn the prospective home owner who is planning to build an *ecologic house.*

STRUCTURAL RESPIRATION THROUGH
THE WALL SECTION

Structural respiration through the wall section is seldom considered to be related to health problems. Clinical ecologists have observed, however, some unusual case histories in this regard. Air tends to travel in unsuspecting pathways. This is caused particularly by an unequal atmospheric pressure between the outside and the inside of the house. Figure 5-1 illustrates one airway that produces unplanned air exchange within a house but that may be unhealthful.

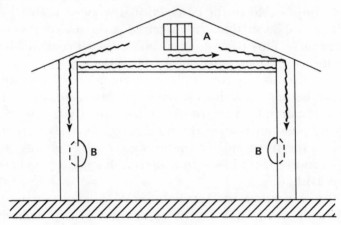

A IS A VENT GRILL IN THE ATTIC
B INDICATE ELECTRIC OUTLETS

Figure 5-1.

Point A in Figure 5-1 is a vent grill in the attic that allows outside air to start its journey on the way into the house. Points B are indicative of electrical convenience outlets. The air from the attic passes downward through the wall section and enters the room through the electrical outlets. On a windy day one need only place the back of his hand near an electrical outlet and feel the cold blast to confirm this phenomenon.

The air that exists at point *b* as illustrated in Figure 5-1, is frequently harmful to the hypersensitive person. This is due to the ecology of the wall cavity. The warmth from the inside and the chill from the outside meet in the wall cavity. The reaction between the two temperatures tends to condense the moisture within the air in the wall cavity. The absence of sunlight in the wall cavity allows mold growth. This sort of pollution in the patient's domestic environment has frustrated many a physician as he has attempted to discover the source of the trouble. The case history from Linda Clark, which was mentioned in the previous chapter, attests to the complexity of this problem.

The question is posed, "How shall we prevent the incitements caused by structural respiration?" Total prevention is probably impossible in the conventional wood-structure house shell. It would seem that the preferred construction would be solid masonry. This can be accomplished with cement blocks, poured-in-place concrete, or adobe blocks.

If one resorts to masonry wall-structure, a need for adequate insulation becomes a serious problem. There is no commercial insulating material on the market that is totally free from the outgassing phenomenon. If the insulating materials were to be applied on the inner side of the masonry wall, the outgassing from this source would be seriously troublesome to a hypersensitive individual.

The use of masonry shell structure calls for engineering specifications not now in use. Several principles suggest themselves. Firstly, the outside face of the masonry wall would need to be completely sealed. A material marketed under the name of Thoroseal®, with a low outgassing capacity, might be utilized for this purpose. Secondly, the insulation applied to the sealed wall facing might be of various types. In some areas application of aluminum foil may be adequate. In colder localities the foil may need to be fortified with a batt type of insulation or sprayed-on polyfoam insulation. The insulation material would need to be veneered with weather-resisting material.

The foregoing, suggested construction is so novel that it may be impossible to find a construction contractor in a given community who would be willing to undertake such a project. In such a case one might apply aluminum foil on both sides of the masonry wall and thereby simplify the application of the veneering materials. The inside wall could be plastered, which would minimize the hazards of outgassing.

In the southwestern part of our nation, the author of this chapter has observed successful use of adobe and stucco veneering. This type of construction, if reinforced with aluminum foil insulation on the inner side of the shell structure, might prove adequate in about 75 percent of the continental United States.

It should be pointed out that adobe is not considered a good insulator in the building trade. Actually, adobe is a good heat sink. It absorbs heat, and when the input source is discontinued, the stored heat in adobe radiates into the surrounding space. This characteristic of adobe has provided comfortable living spaces to southwesterners for many centuries without additional insulation. This experience has implied to uninformed persons that adobe is an excellent insulating material. If its true character is understood, however, it would broaden the application of adobe.

It should be emphasized that clinical observation indicates that there are no foolproof materials for the hypersensitive individuals. Consequently, the foregoing discussion suggests that structural applications must be accepted with reservations. No adequate research exists to assure that any type of shell structure will completely prevent a chemical reaction in the acutely hypersensitive person.

WINDOW ECOLOGY

The window unit of the wall structure contributes in a unique way toward the problem of indoor pollution. Firstly, most windows leak air. Secondly, windows permit the sunlight to overheat drapes, which causes outgassing. On the other hand, if the drapes are open, then the sun's rays fall on the carpet, which also induces outgassing. Since the outgassing impinges on the hypersensitive individual's health, it is important to minimize the effect associated with the window unit in the wall structure.

Several things can be done to minimize the environmental impact of the windows. The usual single-glass window should be substituted with a double-glazed unit. The clear glass should be replaced with a solar heat-filtering glass. The wood frame, which requires troublesome refinishing, can be replaced with metal frame (especially aluminum). Furthermore, the joint between the window frame and the wall section should be thoroughly caulked before the window is set in place. This procedure is superior to the usual dry-set window installation. In addition to the foregoing window-induced pollution, the problem can be minimized by proper screening, venetian blinds, and the use of nongassing drapes. Metal blinds and linen drapes are conducive to the need in question. Screens allowing one-way visibility tend to deflect the sun's direct impact, which will also minimize the outgassing phenomenon in regard to the window unit. Lastly, a long overhang of the roof line will add substantially to minimizing the sun's impact, without eliminating the desired natural light.

DOOR ECOLOGY

The major contaminating effect from doors is the outside air infiltration and the outgassing of the finishing materials. The latter can be overcome easily by use of metal doors with baked-on enamel finish.

There are many styles of metal doors on the market with attractively simulated wood grain appearance. Therefore, the usual objection to metallic appearance has been eliminated. Furthermore, the fire safety of metal doors is superior to that of wood doors.

The outside-air infiltration around doors is ecologically the most troublesome factor. It has been stated repeatedly in this book that the polluted outside air tends to enhance the indoor pollution. Consequently, it is imperative to prevent as much of the infiltration as possible. This can be done in several ways with the door situation.

Weather-stripping is the simplest way to minimize air leaks around the door. There are several basic types of sealing strips. Some are rubberoid materials, some are fabric strips, and some are springy metallic types. Unfortunately, this method of stopping outdoor-air infiltration is seriously limited and inefficient.

The storm-door approach to air infiltration is considered a major improvement over the weather-stripping method. Mostly, this is psychological instead of real. The common aluminum-frame storm door is too frail for a tight closure. It tends to be a slamming hazard on windy days, but the air infiltration is hardly less around the inside door because of the loose closure around the storm door.

In this respect the British people can teach the Americans a lesson. They have developed an effective air interlock. They call it a vestibule. In our society this approach to preventing the invasion of our living rooms by the great outdoors has not been popular. For the hypersensitive individual the use of a vestibule is highly commendable.

The vestibule structure provides a stable anchor for a solid second door. Most importantly, the vestibule creates a type of air-pressure lock. After the first door is closed, the space in the vestibule creates minimal air-pressure imbalance with the larger house space. This prevents huge air volume infiltration when a person is exiting or entering, as well as creating a tight block between the outdoors and the indoors at all other times.

SUMMARY

With reference to the shell-structure ecology, various unique suggestions can be made. The walls can be of masonry materials. The walls can be insulated on the outside instead of inside an inner cavity. The windows can be solar-filtering glass with airtight double-glazed glass. The attic can be power vented, and the doors can be made more effective with the construction of a vestibule. However a person may feel about adding a vestibule to his house, ecologically it is a sound practice and is highly recommended for hypersensitive individuals.

Considering the preceeding discussion of developing airtight shell structures for homes, one might ask the question, "Where will a householder obtain a supply of clean air?" This is a legitimate question that will be answered elsewhere in this book. Suffice it to say that in areas with heavy outdoor pollution, the air that is supplied through a controlled intake must be purified. Furthermore, in areas with tolerable outdoor air, one still must consider the need for air purification because of internally generated air pollution. The details of air treatment through the depollution process is discussed more extensively in other chapters.

Chapter 6

OUTFITTING THE INSIDE

CASIMIR M. NIKEL

THE term *outfitting* in the title of this chapter applies to two concepts. One concept is that of supplying apparel for a special occasion, which implies a process of covering. The other concept is that of supplying equipment and materials for a specific usage, such as an expedition, a trade, or a business enterprise.

The concept of covering will deal with the floor, wall, and ceiling surfaces on the inside of individual rooms in an ecologic house. Covering materials for this purpose are generally termed carpeting, tiling, paneling, plastering, drywall, paints, shellacs, varnishes, sheeting materials, and masonry materials. The latter need not be part of the plastering process. It can involve tile laying, brick or stone masonry, or pouring of concrete, terrazzo, etc. The selection of the most tolerable material, as well as the process of its application, is extremely important for the hypersensitive person. Therefore, detailed attention must be given to these aspects of constructing an ecologic house. This discussion will review these matters with appropriate explanations later in this chapter.

The concept of equipping will deal with furnishings. On first thought, furnishings suggest articles of furniture only. If one would make an inventory, however, of all the physical articles in a house, the result would be astonishing. It would include machinery as well as furniture. For example, one hardly ever thinks of machinery being confined to the house, yet modern technology surprisingly crams a house with numerous items of machinery. Daily we use equipment of this class for purposes of cooling, heating, cleaning, ventilating and entertaining.

Significantly, it should be recognized that some of the furniture and equipment creates pollution. Such pollution consists

53

of *thermal*, radioactive, gaseous, and other harmful ambient input. Clinical ecology has firmly established the harmful effects from many of the household furnishings. Probably the most recent awareness of harmful effect from furnishings has been the discovery of outgassing by synthetic fabrics and upholstering materials (1).

In view of the numerous polluting furnishings and structural materials found in the modern home, it is important to explore all possibilities of avoidance by elimination and substitution wherever it is feasible to do so. Consequently, detailed discussion of furnishings will be treated as a separate item in this chapter.

Outfitting is not the only term that needs some explanation for the discussion in this chapter. The terms floor, walls, and ceiling are much more complex than common usage implies. The meaning of each, which this author will apply to them, will be limited in scope.

To the casual observer, a house is a singular structure. In technical reality, however, it consists of many components and subassemblies. A floor, for example, consists of girders, joists, subflooring, and a top veneer that may be any one of many commonly used materials. The floor, therefore, is an independent component of the whole house. It is designed and constructed according to the purpose it serves. The foundation floor, for example, can be reinforced concrete in a split-level house, while the floor for the top-level rooms in the same house might be a wood structure of girders, joists, and two veneers. What is true of the floor, as an independent component, is similarly true of the wall structure and the ceiling structure. The factors of the walls and ceiling will be discussed by others in this book; consequently, it is necessary to emphasize that the use of the terms walls and ceilings in this chapter will deal exclusively with the veneering process and the veneering materials. It is this author's concerned hope that there will be no confusion about the use of his terms regarding the floor, wall, and ceiling factors.

FINISHING THE INSIDE

The three major surfaces requiring finishing inside a room

consist of the already mentioned floor, walls, and ceiling. After the shell of a house is completed, the inside finishing starts with veneering of the substructure. The veneers are durable surface materials and are mostly undecorated on the walls and ceiling. The floor veneers generally are materially different from the remaining room surfaces. Also, the variety of floor veneers is probably more complex than that of the walls and ceiling, although notedly in recent years wall decors of synthetic derivation have proliferated in the building trades. Without arguing about the relative predominance of these veneers, we shall begin our discussion under two subheadings, i.e. flooring and wall and ceiling veneers.

Floor Materials

For numerous reasons the earliest innovations in the building industry have been the floor veneers. Within the last decade it has become popular to carpet floors throughout the entire house in new construction. It has also become difficult, for economic reasons, to avoid synthetic-fiber carpeting. Consequently, the modern homes have become intolerable, because of outgassing, to most of the hypersensitive persons (2). Because of the recency in this development, many patients do not receive the proper diagnosis; therefore, they are doomed to an interminable time of chronic misery. Ecologic clinicians have firmly established, however, that outgassing of synthetic fibers is harmful to the hypersensitive patient. A survey was made of the physicians who hold membership in the Society for Clinical Ecology in order to provide the most recent facts on this subject.

Fifteen various floor-veneering materials were selected and presented in a listing for the physicians to consider. Seventy percent of the respondents expressed preference for hardwood and terrazzo floor veneers, 60 percent preferred quarry tile, 45 percent indicated concrete as their choice, and 5 percent chose slate for the floor covering. The remaining veneers were incriminated as harmful to hypersensitive patients.

Although wood evoked a high preference, it is still suspect for the hypersensitive. It was noted that *terpene woods* are particularly troublesome. Also, the processing of wood materials often renders them troublesome to hypersensitivities. The offensiveness of woods is sufficiently frequent that it is recommended that any hypersensitive person should be tested for the particular hardwood contemplated for usage. Most importantly it should be noted that all types of synthetic materials in carpeting, plastic tile, and polyfoam rubberoid paddings were rejected by these knowledgeable physicians.

From the foregoing it would seem that masonry and natural materials are the ecologically preferred floor veneers. For the fastidious homemaker this poses an austere environment. To create cheerfulness, cotton-platted (hook-weave) throw rugs can be used. Such rugs lend themselves to dusting outside the house. They can also be washed frequently, especially in the larger-size machines at neighborhood washeterias.

One important aspect of wood for floor veneering must be brought out besides probable hypersensitivity to the wood stock itself — the pollution associated with glue and petrochemical adhesives. This makes inlaid flooring, for example, suspect. The use of glues in manufacturing of the inlay woodblocks may disqualify the original acceptable wood stock. Also, the use of cements for installation of inlay woodblocks may disqualify an inlaid-wood flooring. Hopefully, the reader of this discussion will also become aware that any form of plywood is suspect. The adhesives utilized during manufacturing of plywoods may disqualify a compatible original wood stock.

From the foregoing it can be concluded that the use of concrete, terrazzo, slate, mortar-set quarry tile, and kiln-fired mosaic tile are the material choices for floor veneering. It should not be assumed, however, that this will completely assure that the hypersensitive will not react to such materials. The various mixtures of mortar-setting materials hold a high potential for intolerance. Many masonry cements are not virginally pure. Some trace contaminants might still disturb a critically hypersensitive person. In fact, one physician reported having treated a patient for susceptibility to concrete pollution. This writer has personally experienced some of this in situations where crumbled concrete dust is within tight enclosures.

However, normally stable concrete materials are not bothersome.

Terrazzo and tempered concrete are the most preferred of all masonry veneers for an ecologic house. The masonry tiles would provide the possibility of bacteria and mold growth in the porous mortar joints; therefore, such floor veneer would be classed as second-best. The wood veneer has problems with bacteria and dust collection in joints. Also, the problem with varnish and shellac for finishing of wood floors may preclude the use of wood. Personally as a chemically susceptible person, the author has found all of the materials discussed in this paragraph to be tolerable, with the exception of carpeting. However, based on his historically long experience with personal hypersensitivity plus the research in this field, the recommended material for the ecologically acceptable floor is terrazzo or some similar masonry material, such as slate, quarry tile or kiln-fired mosaic tile.

Wall and Ceiling Materials

The choice of a suitable wall and ceiling veneer is of prime importance, partly because of cost, but mostly because once it is installed, replacement is most difficult. Replacement of wall veneers is not accomplished as readily as discarding offensive drapery or throw rugs. Yet the unhealthfulness of wall and ceiling veneers has a high potential to trouble a hypersensitive person.

Of ten groups of materials used for wall and ceiling veneering and decor submitted to clinical ecologists for their findings, only one of the ten materials was not incriminated as harmful. The singular, not-incriminated, material is ceramic tile. It should be noted here that the ceramic tile must be set in masonry grout. Under no circumstances should chemical adhesives be utilized for setting ceramic tile in dwellings to be occupied by hypersensitive persons. Other commonly utilized wall veneers with minimum incompatibility are troweled plaster, gypsum board, and wood paneling. All three, however, pose disadvantages for the hypersensitive person.

Plaster, Drywall, and Wallpaper

The principal problem with plaster and drywall veneers is the necessary decor material. If wallpaper is used for decorating, the required adhesive might turn out to be a harmful incitant. It is also conceivable that the dyes in the wallpaper decoration can cause trouble. The use of plastic sheeting as a decor veneer for the wall must be done only on advice of the ecologic clinician. Experience suggests that it is unlikely that many hypersensitive persons can tolerate plastic materials over a prolonged period during the heating season. The outgassing from such sheeting may be minimal on the perimeter walls; however, the inside supporting walls tend to build up temperatures high enough to cause harmful levels of pollution by the outgassing process. If the decorative sheeting wall materials are avoided by painting, then special precautions must be taken, which will be discussed in another place of this book.

Gypsum board is an attractive wall veneer because of its economy. For quite some time it was considered acceptable for the dwellings of hypersensitive persons, especially if the joints between the panels were sealed with troweled plaster. Sealing these joints with tape requires incompatible adhesives; therefore, ecologic clinicians recommended strongly the omission of taping.

Recently a special problem has been discovered in connection with gypsum board. A Dallas, Texas physician observed that the drywall veneer in his office was seemingly causing him serious physical discomfort. After careful testing to confirm the source of troublesome pollution, samples of the wallboard were submitted to a professional ecologist who is trained as a pollution analyst. The gypboard samples were disassembled and the plaster portion was unincriminated. The paper binder, however, was causing harmful reactions. A search of wholesalers in the area indicated that some production lots of gypsum board were troublesome, while other production lots were free of the harmful pollution. At the time of this writing, drywall veneers must be considered as an undependable source of material for an ecologic house.

Wood Paneling

Probably the more desirable wall and ceiling veneer is virgin, solid wood paneling. Despite its higher initial cost, it provides advantages over the plaster-type veneers, but its application must avoid use of adhesives. Nailing the panels to the wall studs is the preferred method of applying solid hardwood paneling. Another alert that should be included here pertains to the wood itself. Plywood panels contain adhesives that hold the top finishing layer to a sublayer of cheaper wood. Often the sublayer may be made up of compressed sawdust, which is highly impregnated with adhesives. Such paneling is generally fabricated at low temperatures. Most often it is air-dried. The result is an outgassing when the installed paneling is warmed by the house heating system. This produces troublesome inciteful pollution for the hypersensitive person.

It appears from the foregoing that wood veneers for the walls and ceilings should possess several characteristics: (1) that highly emanating terpene wood stock is not permissable; (2) that hardwood stock is preferred, i.e. birch, oak, walnut, ash, hickory, maple, and cherry species are most often tolerated by hypersensitivies; (3) that the wood wall-veneer should consist of solid virgin wood stock — no plywood is acceptable; (4) that more important than any other imperative is the decor finishing material applied to the wood paneling. Preferably the paneling should be factory prefinished, and the finish should be applied under high temperatures and not air-dried. Paneling treated in this fashion is designated as such in the manufacturer's specification literature.

Concern about the cost of solid impregnated wood paneling for wall veneers has caused this writer to explore alternate materials. Recently, compressed particulate wood materials have been produced, which might be tolerated by many hypersensitive persons. Marlite® is such a material. It is prefinished, and it is cured with temperatures exceeding 200°F. This renders it more stable chemically at household comfort temperatures and probably more tolerable to most hypersensitive persons. Exploration with other hypersensitive ecologists suggests Marlite, Formica®* and one or two other brands of hard-finish wall paneling are more tolerable than most man-made veneers that are produced to simulate the appearance of virgin wood. Hopefully also such substitutes for virgin wood will cost less.⟩

Masonry

Up to this point all the wall and ceiling veneers have been considered as minimally suitable. There are some materials that are more fully acceptable. In the predominant American culture, they are considered, however, as incompatible with domestic use. Their use has been relegated principally to commercial and institutional applications. All these materials belong to the masonry family:

1. Kiln-fired ceramic tile
2. High temperature fired brick†
3. Precast concrete paneling
4. Native field and ledge stone

With imagination, attractive wall patterns can be developed. Warmth to such walls can be added by alternating sections of wood paneling with hanging tapestries, such as Indian native-made wool drapes and wool rugs. Again, it must be noted that such tapestries must not be colored with commercial petrochemical dyes. Another warning seems in order — all tile and stone must be set in mortar. The use of synthetic adhesives might render a house intolerable to a hypersensitive person.

In the case of veneering the walls with masonry materials, the ceiling can be covered with contrasting materials. It might consist of troweled plaster or of wood paneling. The paint required for finishing the plaster, however, is a problem. At this point it seems appropriate to briefly review the painting of inside house surfaces.

Paints

At the time of this writing, there is no paint on the market

---

*T.G. Randolph states that Formica is rarely incriminated as an incitant to the chemically susceptible person.
†It is important that the brick not be treated chemically after it has been kiln fired.

identified as *hypoallergenic*. This contrasts with the situation a decade ago. Exploration with the research laboratories of major paint manufacturers has produced some surprising sidelights in regard to paints. The federal government has alerted the industry, according to some reliable sources, that paints may become classified in the category of prescription medications. This seems hardly feasible; nevertheless, this information is from a responsible source.

One wonders why there is such a drastic proposal by federal authorities. When the ecology of petrochemically derived materials is properly understood, such action by the government seems within reasonable limits.

The paint industry has tried to produce a water-based paint to counteract the ill effects of petrochemically derived paints. This worked but a short time. It was discovered that water-based paints produced molds. So, fungicide was added, which makes the paint intolerable to many hypersensitive persons. And so the merry-go-round goes around, and no one can predict its effect in a given case of hypersensitivity to paints.

Analyzing the situation relative to the hypersensitive and his paints, some safeguards do exist. An easy test to determine tolerance consists of painting a paddle and sleeping on it after thorough drying. For the most dependable results, the paddle should not be put on the bottom side of the pillow. If the paddle is too uncomfortable inside the pillow case, it can be wrapped in a couple thicknesses of a towel. But maximum exposure to the nostrils should be attempted while the paddle is warmed by the side of the face and head during sleep.

If none of the brands of paint tested are tolerable, then there is only one alternative. The plaster should be left its natural color. When it needs cleaning, a skim coat of plaster can be troweled over the original coat. Of course in the case of impregnated wood paneling, the whole business of testing for paint tolerance should be carried out by the physicians.

FURNISHING THE INSIDE

Earlier in this chapter it was alluded that outfitting involved equipping. Within the context of the ecologic house, equipping will deal with the furniture and appliances normally found within a modern home. This, of course, is no easy subject to discuss, since almost no records of definitive *empirical* research can be found on this subject. Ecologic clinicians have observed, however, a tight relationship between certain types of furnishings and their hypersensitive patients. Their lectures and writings are the only reliable basis on which conclusive decisions can be made.

Clinical evidence has established that chemical emanation from synthetic padding and cushion coverings of furniture can be harmful to a hypersensitive person (3). Doctor Randolph reports numerous instances of patients becoming ill "from sitting on sponge rubber or plastic upholstered furniture; from sleeping on sponge rubber mattresses or sponge rubber pillows [commonly advertised as hypoallergenic material] or beds in which mattresses and pillows were covered with plastic encasings" (4). There is no doubt that "the most common harmful synthetics in our homes are furnishings" (5). The most obvious polluting furnishings within living space are newly installed carpets (5). Their outstanding rivals are the gas-fired cooking ranges and gas-fired furnaces (6). Doctor Igho H. Kornblueh, chief of the department of medicine and rehabilitation at the University of Pennsylvania, is quoted to have said, after considering the indigenous pollution discussed heretofore, that "the air inside an average home is actually more polluted than the air outside it." How do we combat this indoor pollution, the source of which is the indispensable furniture and appliances? Principally by avoidance, substitution, and by medical supportive care. Medical supportive care will be discussed by others. Our attention here will be directed to avoidance and substitution.

Avoidance of Incitants

Avoidance involves various approaches. Elimination of all plastics and synthetic fibers is one important method. On first thought this seems impossible. For example, it has been reported that one major chemical manufacturer displayed a room that had been stripped of all furnishings containing petro-

chemical materials in a television ad. The only item left in the
room was a wood rocking chair. Presumably, this kind of ex-
hibit intended to affirm our dependence on petrochemicals.
Yet, this is a simplistic approach.

/Too often very good and chemically acceptable items of
available furniture are overlooked — namely, steel with baked
enamel finish. Wrought iron furniture is another example.
Hardwood furniture, finished with well-seasoned varnish, is
also commonly available and generally tolerated by the hypersensitive person. For living room use such furniture can be
cushioned with custom-made pads. Such pads are to be made
up of coils in wired frames and covered with cotton felt and
cotton *ticking.* /

One warning regarding the choice of ticking should be mentioned — it should not be decorated with petrochemical dyes.
Also, frequently *sizing* materials are troublesome to the hypersensitive in the ticking. Sizing can be washed out before the
material is applied to the cushion pads. In any event all ticking
should be tested for tolerance before approval of its use is given
to the upholsterer, who by necessity must fabricate the custom-
made pads.

Testing of ticking is rather simple. A swatch of the material
can be pinned onto an inside garment and worn that way for
several days. A week or two with more than one swatch is not
an excessive test. The swatch should be located on the chest
area near the collar in order to create inhalant exposure as well
as direct skin contact exposure.

Another test can be made by sitting on a large piece of the
test material. This is best evidence if the material is folded at
least into four thicknesses and is large enough to show about a
6-inch strip on each side of the sitting hypersensitive person.
The sitting test should be of at least one-hour duration on each
of several occasions. This can be done during leisurely television viewing at the end of the day.

One more method of testing tolerance for an intended ticking
material is to sleep on it. The pillow can be wrapped in the
ticking material, and the hypersensitive person should sleep on
it several nights if tolerance is to be confirmed. If symptoms are
detected immediately, then two or three nights should be al-

lowed to pass and a repeat test should be made to affirm that it is the ticking that causes the reaction. If the bothersome symptoms persist, then the ticking should be laundered in soap solution to which tolerance has been established previously, and the test should be repeated as outlined. The test, after the ticking is laundered, will establish if a person is sensitive to something else than the sizing. The "something else" might be either the dye or the cotton stock itself. To prove which is the case in such situations requires the expertise of an ecologic clinician. If a patient is sensitive to either petrochemical dyes or the cotton stock, it is imperative that he obtain medical services.

After tolerance for the ticking and the felt padding is established, the upholsterer can be authorized to fabricate the coil-spring cushions. He should be warned never to try to improve the outer surface appearance by covering the felt with any kind of plastic material before enclosing the cushion with the acceptable ticking.

It might be peremptorily stated that testing for tolerance to the cotton felt, which is used by the upholsterer, is similar to tolerance testing for the ticking material. A sample of felt material can be placed in a pillow case for the sitting and sleeping test in order to keep it intact.

The foregoing suggestions are only a partial avoidance technique. In all probability in cases of extreme hypersensitivity, avoidance by elimination of petrochemicals in the domiciliary environment may still be inadequate. In such instances depollution of the air may become imperative (7).

Another technique of avoidance involves sanitation. Most cotton and wool fabrics used by humans develop molds and mites. These can be avoided by washing, by airing, and by sunning. The latter technique was commonly utilized by our forebears. In rural areas a few homemakers still sun such items as mattresses. Urban dwellers find this procedure inconvenient. A substitute technique to sunning is to expose the mattress and furniture cushions to the rays of an infrared lamp. Pillows, on the other hand, can be tumble-dried in a laundry drier about once each week for similar effect to sunning. Also, all linen that has been stored temporarily in the closet should be tumble-dried before using it on the bed.⁷

Another sanitizing technique involves vacuuming such items as mattresses and furniture cushions. The preferred vacuum machine should pass the discharge air through water, not through the conventional dry filter bag.

Substitution for Incitants

Substitution, although more easily achieved, involves greater limitations than avoidance as a technique of combatting indoor pollution. Substituting furniture that is heavily upholstered with synthetic fabrics with metal and hard-finished wood furniture has been mentioned under avoidance techniques. The biggest potential for substitution is in the area of fabrics and wall decor items, as well as in the area of appliances. Substitutes for synthetic fabrics include the following: cotton, wool, silk, and cellular *rayons*.* These substitutions can be included in items of drapery, carpeting, bed linens, tapestry, etc.

Probably the most difficult area for substitution of synthetics involves wearing apparel. Cotton clothing seldom can maintain the beauty of synthetic garments. Maintenance of cotton is also more difficult, but for the hypersensitive person who is suffering from intolerable symptoms that are induced by synthetic fabrics it is a choice of beauty or suffering. It is presumed that some attractiveness can be sacrificed to obtain relief from chronic ailments.

Too often it is assumed that natural products can be tolerated by all hypersensitives. This is not a valid assumption. Patients are on record who reacted violently to cotton materials but were tolerant to synthetic fabrics. Opinionated individuals may cavil about this, but empirical methodology cannot disregard the occurrence of actual phenomenon. Clinically observed deviation from natural materials also confirms the foregoing theory. It is commonly accepted by allergy specialists that some patients are

---

*Cellular rayons are made generally from wood fibers. A warning is appropriate because a whole battery of rayons now exist that are of petrochemical derivation, which of course are taboo for hypersensitives.

sensitive to wool, which is a natural product. Sensitivity to silk also has been established clinically (8). The question may be raised, "If sensitivity exists to silk and wool, then why not to cotton?"

If substitutes from the family of natural products is not tenable, it seems important that no hypersensitive should depend on his own judgment in determining which clothing fabrics are acceptable. Such a decision should be made under the guidance of an astute physician.

Decor substitutes are extremely limited. If a person is sensitive to wall pictures and paintings, a few substitutes are available, principally such materials as china dishes, decorative (adhesive free) mirrors, metal plaques, and shelf objects made of glass, silver, gold, brass, ceramics, etc. Persons hypersensitive to ink and color dyes would be advised to refrain from decorating rooms with shelf-displayed books. Too often these exposures are overlooked.

The most difficult substitution involves appliances. Generally gas-fired ranges, furnaces, refrigerators, and other illumination and heating items that utilize gas can be substituted with electrical counterparts if it is established that the hypersensitive person is intolerant to natural gas. Some hypersensitives, however, are intolerant to pollution created by electrical refrigerator motors, electrical transformers, electrical air cleaners, and sound transmission equipment, such as radios and television circuitry. One of the authors in this book reports sensitivity to the latter two items. In his case it is necessary to exhaust the heated air out of the radio and *television* sets by fan-driven ventilation directly to the outside atmosphere.

Other forms of pollution from electrical equipment that are hazardous, besides *Glyptal*® fumes, is reported by Taub (9). One such pollutant is ozone, and another is radiation. Research evidence reveals that ozone corresponds highly with certain types of cancer and with a hypersensitive respiratory effect. Substituting electrical appliances indiscriminately for gas appliances, therefore, may be worse for the individual than the original problem.

When appropriate testing establishes that substitution with electrical appliances is not feasible, isolation is the only alternative. The appliance must be placed in an isolated, remote utility room. The utility room must be equipped with airtight doors that lead to the living area. Such a room must be provided with direct ventilation to the outside, so that accumulated pollution will not rush into the living area when entrance into the utility room is made. It is evident that when substitution is impossible, isolation is the only means of avoidance.

By now the layman who is afflicted with hypersensitivity, and who has waded through the foregoing, must surely feel confused and doubtful about the feasibility of creating an ecologic house. If this is true, it only proves how complex the technology of clinical ecology is and how important it is for a hypersensitive person to resort to the medical services of a physician who is skilled in these matters. A final word of advice to the hypersensitive person who is seeking to establish a tolerable environment within his home is to find a competent physician and an experienced environmental consultant as his trusty guides in the everlasting struggle for ecological health.

BIBLIOGRAPHY

1. Randolph, Theron G.: *Human Ecology and Susceptibility to the Chemical Environment.* 4th ed. Springfield, Thomas, 1972, pp. 25, 50, 113.
2. Nikel, Casimir M.: *Breathing for Survival.* 1st ed. Hicksville, New York, Exposition, 1975, pp. 19, 62, 68, 74, and 75.
3. Taub, Harold J.: *Keeping Healthy in a Polluted World.* 1st ed. New York, Har-Row, 1974, p. 221.
4. Randolph, *Human Ecology and Susceptibility to the Chemical Environment*, pp. 12, 20, 45, 46, 57, and 107.
5. Nikel, *Breathing for Survival*, pp. 19, 55, 73.
6. Heiman, S.J.: *Before You Forget your Heating Worries*, a monograph #1964-060667. Available from Intertherm, Inc., 3800 Park Avenue, St. Louis, Missouri 63110.
7. Nikel, *Breathing for Survival*, pp. 96-99.
8. Randolph, *Human Ecology and Susceptibility to the Chemical Environment*, pp. 12, 34.
9. Taub, *Keeping Healthy in a Polluted World*, pp. 221-224.

Chapter 7

THE ECOLOGY OF HEAT

Casimir M. Nikel

THE relationship of heat to good health has been neglected too long, but gradually information from clinical experience is pointing up the importance of this situation. Louis Pasteur is reported to have observed that the anthrax bacillus had no effect when injected into chickens, but sheep would die when injected with the same vaccine. Investigation established that the body temperature of a chicken is higher than that of sheep, and this provided an intolerable environment for the anthrax bacillus.

More recently Louis Kervran, a French physician and health commissioner, was assigned to investigate the cause of an epidemic of carbon monoxide (CO) poisoning among some construction workers (1). His investigation revealed that the carbon monoxide poisoning was occurring among a group of welders. He surmised that elevation of body temperature could be a cause of the carbon monoxide poisoning.

Testing of carbon monoxide levels in the blood of the welders under investigation indicated that their CO blood levels were lower before work and higher after engaging in welding. Capturing the air at the nostrils during the welding activity established that this was not the source of the offending gas. After considerable tracing, airtight face masks were applied with long hoses to provide control of the air intake. Experimentation established that if the air remote to the hot welding metal was inhaled, no change in blood level of CO occurred. However, if the air intake was directed over the hot metal then the carbon monoxide in the blood level would rise. It is presumed from this experiment that hot air caused a mutation inside the blood stream. Under normal body temperature, carbon dioxide is formed, whereas, when the welders inhaled hot air the mutation resulted in a buildup of carbon monoxide within the blood stream of the welders.

Such incidents as described in the experience of Pasteur and Kervran pinpoint attention to other situations in which application of heat might have an effect on the health of humans. Particular attention has been given to the perennial outbreak of sinus, bronchial, and chest infections each fall when the house is closed up and furnace heat is released into the domiciliary environment. Empirical studies indicate that two conditions develop from furnace heating. The high temperature of the heat exchanger in the furnace produces what is called *fried dust*. This fried dust releases various gases depending on the source of the dust in the air. Also, the improper combustion air mixtures also produce gases harmful to human health. It has been determined by careful investigations that it is the improper applications of heat for the conditioning of the ambient air that relates to the onset of upper respiratory infections during the cold period of each year.

Now heating systems are being so designed that it is possible to overcome the chronic illnesses caused by conventional heating systems. The earliest of such systems is the hydronic convectors heated from a remote boiler. The electric hot-water-without-plumbing system (*Intertherm®*) is a more recent development. The latest systems involve *laminar induction* with the use of a low temperature, remote heat pump and the hot water solar system. Each of the latter two systems is in various experimental stages of development. Hopefully by the time this book is published, production models will be available.

In view of the importance of heat ecology, the editors of this book have requested contributions from authors on the most recently developed heating systems. The electric hot water system has a well-tested history and is most readily available. The laminar heat pump and solar applications are in early stages of development, but because of their potential, they are presented for the reader's consideration. One thing is paramount in consideration of domiciliary heating systems — the operating temperature should be low, and the air movement should be convected by the natural physics of heat and not forced with power-driven fans. If power movement of air is employed, the movement should be of such velocity as not to disturb the microscopic dust within the ambient air. It is considered that each of the systems discussed herein meets both of the two requisite factors of ecologic heat applications.

BIBLIOGRAPHY

1. Kervran, Louis C.: *Biological Transmutations*. Binghampton, New York, Swan House (English version), pp. 16-19.

Chapter 8

THE ECOLOGY OF
ELECTROHYDRONIC HEATING

Sidney J. Heiman

IT is unfortunate to see chronically ill individuals suffering from sensitivity to the contaminants being released into their own home year after year by their own heating systems, most often with no possible chance of relief. It is especially distressing if they have called in a heating specialist who has rejected any chance of a problem of this nature or if they will not admit to themselves this is possible.

In my association with the Society for Clinical Ecology for the past ten years, I was simply astonished the first time that I read Doctor Theron G. Randolph's book entitled *Human Ecology and Susceptibility to the Human Environment* in which he tells about a patient who suffered for thirty years from her exposure to petrochemical contamination caused by heating systems and other appliances. This patient was about to be committed to a mental hospital because her physicians finally concluded that her condition was entirely due to mental problems. Doctor Randolph, upon consultation, discovered her sensitivity to petrochemical contamination. Fortunately this patient was spared from the agony of being placed into an asylum in this way.

Later in discussing the matter with Doctor Randolph, I found that this was not an isolated case. It was difficult for me to believe there were many many cases of this nature which unfortunately were not being treated. To my amazement, Doctor Randolph informed me that 94 percent of all the patients being referred to him from throughout the United States and foreign countries were sensitive in some way to the petrochemicals released by combustion heating systems and other appliances in the home, as well as to the release of gases from the synthetic materials used in the home.

71

Having been in the heating business for over forty-seven years at that time, I found this information most difficult to accept. I was aware that there was some relationship between one's health and the heating system in the home the moment doors and windows were closed for the winter months, but could it really be possible that people were actually that sensitive to combustion gases?

HOW GAS AND OIL FURNACES
POLLUTE THE AIR IN HOMES

The conventional gas heating furnace or boiler is designed to provide a certain volume of heat each time its flame is turned on by the thermostat. The chimney would then naturally be expected to remove the combustion gases as fast as they are generated. The flame operates on and off intermittently, so each time the flame is turned off, the chimney naturally cools off. Because a cold chimney has no draft at all when the fire is started again, there is no way of drawing the burnt gases out through the chimney. If the combustion gases are not removed, however, they smother the fire and cause carbon monoxide, which is deadly toxic. It is for this reason gas furnaces allow these gases to escape into the home, which is done by means of a "draft divertor" until the chimney gets hot enough to start drawing again.

This same type of draft-divertor device is used with gas water heaters and incinerators. The combustion gases are released directly into the home from these devices.

Oil heating systems at the present time have a different arrangement in the form of a draft regulator that naturally serves the same purpose as the draft divertor, and the gaseous petrochemicals of combustion are naturally released into the home in somewhat the same manner.

It's very simple, of course, for anyone to prove for himself how these gases are released into the home. All he needs to do is to stand near the grilled opening at the top-front of the heating system when the thermostat starts the heat and smell these gases spreading out into the house.

He may not be sensitive to these gases, for which he can be most thankful. One physician tells me that the way he tests his patients for sensitivity is to have them breathe the combustion gases from a lighted gas range to determine whether they are sensitive to them.*

If you are sensitive to these gases, however, you can save yourself distress and tremendous expense by doing something about it instead of suffering with constant medical bills, with no positive relief, and with the problem getting no better.

It is not easy for anyone to accept the fact that his heating system is causing his illness. I have conducted hundreds of lectures throughout the United States and Canada, as well as Japan, before engineers, architects, builders, and physicians explaining how homes are being contaminated with their own heating systems, only to discover again and again these same people saying, "It just can't happen to me," or "It's hard to believe that all of the engineers and architects would allow this to happen." Unfortunately, it is true, and unfortunately it is your life and your health that is involved.

HOW OTHER TOXIC POISONS
ARE RELEASED IN THE HOME

While petrochemicals from combustion gases are basically the greatest source of contaminants in the home, the next most important source is that caused by the tiny lint particles from cotton, wool, linen, silk, and plastic materials in the air, which actually become combusted into additional toxic gases as they come into contact with the 450° to 800°F heat exchanger surfaces of furnaces and electric resistance heaters. While a great deal of scientific data is not available as to the extent of this contamination in homes, any person interested in determining the extent to which he is affected can readily test his sensitivity to these gases by breathing the air from a furnace register or by standing directly over an ordinary electric *resistance heater.* Another way is simply to place gauze or tissue on the heat exchanger surface or fire door of any heating system and then see how fast carbonization and combustion accumulate on its surface.

---

*This test should be performed after the patient has been isolated from exposure to fossil fuel contaminants for at least seventy-two hours.

Figure 8-1 will enable you to evaluate the various types of equipment that are causing these air pollution problems in houses.

CHART SHOWING SOURCE OF POLLUTANTS IN THE HOME

Because of the alarming number of people being discovered sensitive to contaminants released by various types of equipment being used in the home, we have been requested to provide a simple method** of enabling the physician as well as home owner to readily identify sources of these problems as listed below:

		*TOXIC COMBUSTION GASES	OIL VAPORS	*TOXIC GASES FROM BURNT LINT	FRIED LINT DUST	UNBALANCED TEMPERATURES	AIR DRAFTS	HIGH NOISE LEVELS	CORROSIVE OZONE	CAUSES:
GAS	Furnaces Space Heaters	① YES	③ YES	② YES	② YES	YES	④ YES	④ YES		1. Released by draft divertors. 2. From contact with high temperature heat exchanger surfaces. 3. From electric motor oil sumps. 4. From operation of blowers.
GAS	Water Heaters Incinerators	① YES								1. Combustion gases released by draft divertors.
GAS	Cook Stoves Ovens	① YES	③ YES	② YES	② YES					1. Combustion gases released into room. 2. From contact with high temperature heat exchanger surfaces. 3. From baking and frying oils.
GAS	Boilers for Central Heating	① YES	③ YES	② YES	② YES			④ YES		1. Combustion gases released by draft divertors. 2. From contact with high temperature heat exchanger surfaces. 3. Oil vapors from electric motor oil sumps. 4. From air locks in radiators.
OIL	Furnaces Space Heaters	① YES	③ YES	② YES	② YES	YES	④ YES	④ YES		1. Combustion gases released when heater starts. 2. From contact with high temperature heat exchanger surfaces. 3. From electric motor oil sumps. 4. From operation of blowers.
OIL	Water Heaters Ranges Incinerators	① YES		② YES	② YES					1. Combustion gases released each time heater starts. 2. From contact with high temperature heat exchanger surfaces.
ELEC-TRIC	Furnaces Space Heaters Heat Pumps		② YES	① YES	① YES		③ YES	③ YES		1. From contact with high temperature heat exchanger surfaces. 2. Oil vapors from electric motor oil sumps. 3. From operation of blowers.
ELEC-TRIC	Range		① YES	② YES	② YES					1. Released from cooking and baking oils. 2. From contact with high temperature heat exchanger surfaces.
ELEC-TRIC	Baseboard Resistance Heat			① YES	① YES	② YES				1. From contact with high temperature heat exchanger surfaces. 2. From chilling between thermostat cycles.
ELEC-TRIC	Baseboard Hot-Water Heat	*L INTERTHERM*								No contaminants released into the home. Hot water provides uniform floor-to-ceiling comfort.
ELEC-TRIC	Cable Ceiling Heat					① YES				1. All heat beams downward, leaving floors underneath furniture cold.
ELEC-TRIC	Motors	① YES						② YES		1. From electric motor oil sumps. 2. From sparks caused by brush-type motors.
FIL-TERS	Electrostatic	② YES	① YES	① YES					① YES	1. From electric sparks when filters are loaded with dirt. 2. From electric motor oil sumps.
FIL-TERS	Fibrous Oil Saturated	① YES								1. Oil vapors circulated into room air.

*   Olsen and his colleagues (1) have studied the gases produced in experimental fires and have demonstrated the presence of hydrogen cyanide, ammonia, sulfur dioxide, hydrogen sulfide, nitrogen, and oxides of nitrogen, in addition to the expected carbon monoxide and carbon dioxide. Several of these gases could be found in rather high concentrations if the nitrogen content of the combustible material was great, as in the case of wool, silk, and nitrocellulos photographic film. These workers pointed out that two processes proceed simultaneously in a fire: combustion, wherein there is sufficient oxygen to support a flame, and pyrolysis, in which extreme heat is present but where the oxygen concentration is too low to support combustion. Pyrolysis occurs to a greater extent as the fire progresses and the available oxygen supply is consumed (2).

**This chart has been developed in collaboration with Guy O. Pfeiffer, M.D., July 10, 1974

E-4098 072274
PRINTED IN U.S.A.

Intertherm Hot Water Electric Heat Division
INTERTHERM INC./3800 Park Avenue/St. Louis, Missouri 63110

Figure 8-1.

Note that hot-water electric-baseboard heat is the only heating method available on the market that does not cause any contamination. To understand why this is possible, it is most essential to know the construction of the equipment and why Intertherm® hot water electric heat is able to perform as it does.

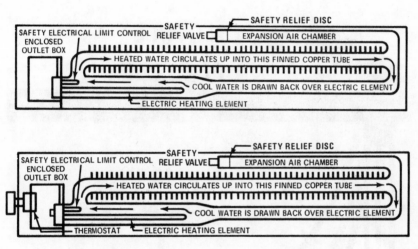

Figure 8-2. Intertherm® hot water electric heat.

Figure 8-2 is a sketch of the inner works of this type of heating equipment. Notice the large tube below at left into which an electric element is welded that connects to a copper tube loop which has fins on the tube above. Water and anti-freeze are introduced into the unit and sealed shut permanently. The electric element then is able to give off its heat as needed.

With Intertherm hot water electric heat, temperatures are maintained so low that it is the only type of electric heater that allows one to insert gauze or tissue paper into its hottest parts without scorching or even yellowing.

Figure 8-3 shows how this method of heating works. The heater is at the base of an outside wall where over 90 percent of the heat required for a room is needed. On the coldest days the water is heated to its maximum temperature to balance the cold air flowing down from outside walls and windows. On a moderate day, however, the water temperature lowers to exactly balance the lesser heat needed, and on a mild day there is just a small amount of heat given off to provide this perfect balance at all times. This is accomplished, of course, by the length of the time the electric heating element stays on. The water-antifreeze solution holds its temperature for over thirty minutes after the electricity is off. In this way the solution's temperature varies with each change in the weather outdoors. As a conse-

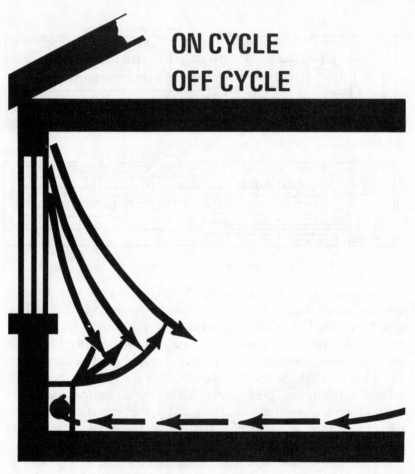

Figure 8-3. Heat distribution.

quence, there is a perfect balance of heat versus cold so that there is no excess heat when very little is needed and too little heat when a great deal is needed.

With the *electric resistance baseboard heaters*, the big problem, of course, is that when the heat goes on, it goes on all the way, and when it goes off, the heat flow stops. On mild days when you need only a little heat, there is too much heat, and the excess heat going to the ceiling runs up heating bills 3.1 percent for every excess degree of temperature that you have at the ceiling. Moreover, this method of heating is very uncomfortable due to the fact that when the heat goes off, it allows the cold air to flow downward and chill the floors even though ceilings are excessively hot.

Manufacturers of furnaces and electric resistance heaters will, of course, never admit it; however, this alternate up-and-down heating will increase bills as much as 30 percent by losing 14° to 16°F to excess ceiling temperatures, even though floors are uncomfortably cold.

An important dimension in heating ecology is not fully recognized yet. It is unbalanced heating, characterized by high temperatures at one part of the body and uncomfortably chilly temperatures at another part. This can cause emotional distress, as well as physical discomfort. If this heat imbalance is supplemented with pollution, which is a related problem in many heating systems, many people experience a great deal of stress. The factors of noisy heating equipment and drafty heat distribution can further aggravate the problem of individuals who are sensitive to the heated air within the home.

The electrohydronic Intertherm system has been designed to minimize problems associated with heating ecology. The system is noiseless. Its pollution output is imperceptible and the distribution of the heat is remarkably uniform. Reliable studies have indicated less than a 5°F temperature rise between floor and ceiling. Many individuals report that they feel a gentle all-over uniform comfort similar to that of being outdoors on a beautiful spring day. The success of the Intertherm system is assured by its use of natural heat convection and continuous heat flow, which is produced by the hot water reserve, even during periods when the thermostat cuts off the electric current to the heater.

In summary, it can be stated that Intertherm heating provides heat ecology resulting in minimum health impairment due to several special features:

1. By operating at approximately 200°F, the microscopic dust in the ambient atmosphere does not become carbonized. The occupants of the room, therefore, are relieved of abrasive fried dust and diffused toxic gases.
2. By allowing normal physics of heat to distribute the warmth throughout the room atmosphere, cleaner air is inhaled. The fan-driven air in other heating systems keeps the house dust in continuous turmoil and suspension. This suspended house dust increases the health hazard for a hypersensitive individual. The slow and continuous saturation of the room air through the Intertherm system eliminates draftiness and minimizes house-dust pollution.
3. By using water to provide continuous heat input a uniformity of heat distribution results. Even when the thermostat cuts off electrical energy input to the heater, the reservoir of heat in the water continues to heat the room. This continuing heat input creates a warm screen in front of the window and outer wall (which is the coldest area of cold infiltration) and thereby protects the floor against an excessive chilling effect. The result is less than 5°F differential between floor and ceiling temperatures. Hypersensitive individuals find this uniform warmth unusually compatible.

BIBLIOGRAPHY

1. Olsen, et al. Cited in Wetherell, H.R.: The occurrence of cyanide in the blood of fire victims. *Journal for Science, II* (2), 1966.
2. Wetherell, H.R.: The occurrence of cyanide in the blood of fire victims. *Journal for Science, II* (2), 1966.

Chapter 9

DESIGN FOR AN ECOLOGIC HEAT PUMP

H. READ MINER

FOR the patient with chemical susceptibility, the use of a groundwater heat pump is preferred over the use of resistance electric heating and conventional air conditioning (1). To achieve the desired results, however, from the groundwater heat pump for the chemically susceptible individual, the heating medium must be a liquid that is circulated inside copper piping which has radiating aluminum fins for most effective heat distribution. The sizing of this equipment must be sufficiently large to operate at 130°F temperature of the liquid and yet maintain comfortable heat levels inside the house when the outdoor atmospheric temperature is below 32°F. Such a system can provide adequate thermal requirements during the coldest periods and give the advantage of borrowed heat at warmer winter periods.

To illustrate the above described design, let us consider the operation of a common household refrigerator, which is used for food storage. Actually it is a heat pump in reverse, as long as it maintains two coils of opposite temperatures. One coil is always hot, and the other coil is always cold. Assuming that the machinery of the domestic refrigerator was reversed so that the Freon® gas was passed through the compressor into the coil inside the refrigerator; this would produce a hot coil inside, and when the Freon returned through the expansion valve to the outside coil, this coil would become cold. Under these conditions the food refrigerator would undergo the same effect the house does when the heat pump transfers outdoor atmospheric heat into the ambient indoor space.

For the chemically susceptible individual, the system described above poses one hazard, namely, the presence of the Freon gas indoors. It is not common knowledge that the tiny leakage of Freon around pipe joints from the air conditioning system can cause serious sickness for the chemically susceptible individual. Clinical ecology has established this to be true. Individuals with such a problem must store gas associated (be it Freon or methane) with air heating or cooling units on the outside of their living quarters. Consequently, to overcome the associated problem, assume that the entire unit that is proposed here was set outside and the hot coil was immersed in a water bath. This water bath could become a reservoir of uncontaminated heat for the chemically susceptible individual during the winter. A similar water bath for the cold coil of the proposed system would serve as a reservoir of coolant during summer weather.

With proper design the above system can produce 14 to 15 Btu per watt of electrical energy consumed, as compared to 3.5 Btu per watt of electricity consumed via the resistance heating system. A similar efficiency (although at a lower ratio) can be obtained with this system during summer operation. The principal ecological advantage of such a system is the ability to heat the ambient indoor space with uncontaminated liquid not exceeding 130°F.

The "heat rejection" factor by the heating and cooling baths mentioned heretofore has been taken into consideration. Reliable calculations suggest that the operating cost of this system will be from one-fourth to one-half the operating cost of a conventional heat pump.

The distribution of the heat inside the house may be through a conventional hydronic convector. It will need to be sized for operation at 130°F of the liquid passing through it, which liquid would be pumped from the water bath outside the house. For cooling purposes the heating convector unit would need a fan to propel the cool air into the ambient space of the house. This would be done at low velocity to minimize the circulation of house dust. Air depollution provisions are included in the thermal distribution units, consequently, maximum ecological advantages would accrue from the system.

The heat-pump principle applied as specified in this chapter has taken into account the availability of equipment, the installation cost versus operating cost offsets, and the maximum ecologic potential for the chemically susceptible individual. In view of escalating energy costs, the amortization of the equipment will be enhanced. Consequently, this concept is confidently presented for its usefulness and feasibility. Anyone desiring to pursue this avenue of conditioning the indoor air for the chemically susceptible individual is invited to communicate with the author of this monograph for details, specifications, and equipment sources.

BIBLIOGRAPHY

1. *Popular Science,* February 1978, pp. 78-82.

Chapter 10

SOLAR HEATING POTENTIAL

JOHN W. ARGABRITE

SOLAR energy heated houses are a probability of the near future. Today they are being constructed with auxiliary backup heating units. These experimental designs can be seen in many areas. Basically, the solar energy heater is found to be of an extremely simple design. The energy is collected from the sun by using an aluminum shield collector that has been painted with a special black or green paint. Among those who are experimenting with this are the architectural planners known as "Sun Mountain Design" (1) (Fig. 10-1). They offer several schematics of solar collectors and "hot air" heaters for sun-supplied energy applications.

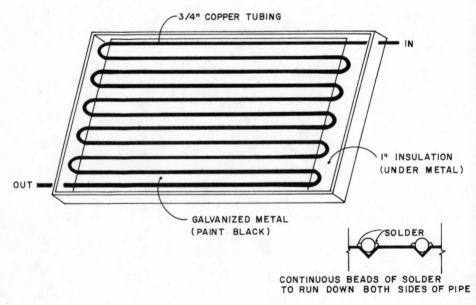

Figure 10-1.

During the day, the sun's heat is stored in a bed of rocks by a simple, active solar furnace or heat collector. Some experimental designs are now using containers of water. The heat is transferred during the night by a fan system in order to keep the indoor space of the home at a constant comfortable temperature.

In a passive solar heating system, the sun's heat can also be conveyed into the home by the way of Thermopane® windows. The walls of the home must be heavily insulated with proper materials. The temperatures of a home that is heated only by way of the Thermopane window (in the Albuquerque, New Mexico area) can vary from 15 to 20°F in a given twenty-four-hour period. During a typical winter twenty-four-hour period, it was found that the indoor temperature would vary from a minimum of 60° to a maximum of 80°F. It must be recognized that this is radiant heat, and, thus, the temperature changes are slow and gradual, so the house atmosphere feels quite comfortable at either extreme.

Tentarelli heats his swimming pool, domestic hot water, and his house space in New Hampshire with a collector fabricated from black aluminum panels and copper pipes molded on opposite sides of the black panels (2) (Fig. 10-1). The storage tank containers are indirectly connected to the sunlight source. Heat transfer from the domestic water is provided by a secondary tank (see Fig. 10-2). Tentarelli also uses a tilting collector to follow the sun to capture the maximum sun energy available on a given day. He estimates that his system has reduced his electrical cost by $120 per year, and it has reduced his propane gas cost for heating the swimming pool by $80 per year.

Solar energy can be used without supplementary energy to heat a swimming pool in the summer because the necessary temperature does not exceed 85°F. Houses, during the winter, need higher water temperatures; however, a combination of solar and electrical systems interconnected to work as a single unit are now on the market. They are reported to accrue substantial fuel cost savings.

Doctor Ronald Winston has perfected a solar concentrator that is able to increase the effect of the incoming sunlight by as much as ten times over the conventional solar collector (3). It does not require a tracking capability to follow the sun

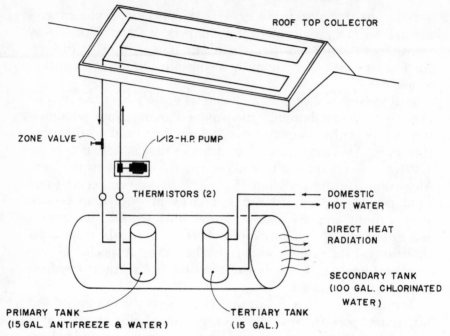

Figure 10-2.

throughout the day. An article entitled "Solar Water Heaters You Can Buy Now" was illustrated and reviewed by Richard Stepler recently (5). Also, International Solarthermics Corporation has developed a solar furnace that can be purchased from stock (6). The major advantage of all these solar systems is the free source of energy and freedom from pollution. The major handicap is their costly initial installation; however, for those who can afford such a system, it is superior to fossil fuel heating systems for the chemically susceptible individual.

Another source of economical and ecologically healthful energy is the windmill-generated electricity. This would be especially true in North Dakota, South Dakota, Minnesota, Wisconsin, and Nebraska. In these states, the prevailing winds are a constant commodity.

It is estimated that the first sailwing electrical generator would be of 5-kw capacity and it "could produce about 12,550 kw hours per year with suitable winds" (7). This could easily serve an average residence if the output was leveled and converted to 60 Hz operation. The author states "that at least 10 kw are needed and more is necessary if your pumps, freezer, refrigerator, and airconditioner obey Murphy's law and decide to hit the line together."

Solar Wind Company makes a unit that produces 6000 w dc/3000 w ac, which was listed at a cost of $10,305 in 1974 (7). The largest system available from this company has a five-day storage capacity and a monthly output of 325 kw per hour in ten-mile-per-hour wind. If more power is necessary, Solar Wind Company suggests combining two Model 6000 Elektron® units with a single set of batteries giving 1000 kwh per month energy supply. Such a combination system costs approximately $18,000 at 1974 prices.

The world's largest windmill generator was built by NASA and is in operation at NASA's Plum Brook Station near Sandusky, Ohio. This mill produces 100 kw, which is estimated to be enough electric power to supply thirty homes with minimum electrical appliances, which would exclude cooking and heating electrically. This project, during its experimental development, is reported to have cost almost $1 million. No cost estimate is available for construction of a single productive unit of this immense dimension.

The estimates of available wind energy, on an annual basis, can be predicted with reasonable reliability. This is contrary to the uncertainty of available petroleum supplies for the long-term future. Consequently, the use of electrical energy generated by windpower has considerable attraction. For the hypersensitive individual, it is doubly attractive in view of its freedom from ambient pollution.

The costs of original solar- and wind-energy equipment currently makes such approaches feasible only to the ultra rich individual. It is estimated that a combination solar heater and wind generator for minimal electrical service would cost approximately $30,000 for a house of 1,500 square feet of floor space. Anything less than this would need supplemental energy, either from the electrical utility company or gas company. However, as it was stated in the opening remarks of this chapter, solar homes are a general possibility in the future, although they may not be economically feasible at present standards and costs.

BIBLIOGRAPHY

1. Price, Travis: Solar homes. *Popular Science,* December 1976, pp. 95-98, 142-143.
2. Moran, Edward: Focusing collectors. *Popular Science,* December 1976, pp. 60-61.
3. Fisher, Arthur: Solar concentrator. *Popular Science,* June 1976, p. 50.
4. Moran, Edward: Photovoltaic cells. *Popular Science,* June 1976, p. 74.
5. Stepler, Richard: Solar water heaters. *Popular Science,* May 1976, pp. 105, 37-38.
6. International Solarthermics Corp., Box 397, Nederland, Colorado 80466.
7. Lindsley, E.F.: Wind power. *Popular Science,* July 1974, pp. 54-59, 34-35. *Solar Wind Company, East Holden, Maine 04429.*

Chapter 11

ECOLOGY OF THE INDOOR AIR

Guy O. Pfeiffer

THERMAL comfort control of the living, sleeping, and working areas supplied with a minimal amount of pollution has been discussed in preceding chapters. The *Oasis* also aids in offering a less contaminated indoor area. However, no matter how precise we attempt to be in the cleanliness of the indoor air, we often find that we are breathing air loaded with pollutants. We must reduce these incitants by filtration.

Laws are being designed to reduce pollution of the outside air, but too little effort has been made in controlling air quality inside the building. Many manufacturers and retail outlets are now beginning to advertise that one should install a filter because increasing air pollution has reduced the availability of outside air that is sufficiently clean to be used for ventilation purposes.

Indoor air pollution must be reduced if we are to enjoy the comfort required for optimal health. In the past few years, more concern for health has been evidenced by the heating, cooling and filtration industry. In the September 6, 1971 issue of *Air Conditioning, Heating and Refrigeration News* magazine appeared a reprint of an article entitled "Importance of Outside Air in Home Heating Systems." It recalled the premise that outside air entered the house of yesteryear through cracks around the windows and doors, through open spaces left during constructions, etc. It further told how the modern contractor, by using newer construction materials such as plastics and vapor barriers, is producing a tighter house. Therefore, air ducts supplying outside air to the furnace are required to balance the oxygen requirements of the heating system. Some buildings require that outside air be brought into the building in order to dilute the indoor pollution, as evidenced by stale air odors. Thus, we arrive at this premise: Indoor air pollution is worse than outdoor air pollution because indoor air has the combination of outdoor air pollution and the pollution produced within the structure.

How are we to reduce the indoor air pollution in order to improve the health of the individual? Removal, or rather major reduction, of the pollutive factors is the end result; however, why produce the pollutants and then improve the methods to remove them? Why not produce as few as possible and then reduce (within feasibility) the few that are produced?

FILTRATION

One way to lower the residual indoor air pollution is through filtration; however, filters are not without potential danger. Poor engineering on the part of the designer of the system, frequent changes made by the building owner and operator, or even negligent or damaging maintenance procedures on the part of maintenance personnel are responsible for the many problems. Comfort engineers have reported that they have found that moisture and dust and sometimes the filter media itself are food for bacteria. Colonies grow. Some of them slough off and end up on the coils in the ductwork and on the face of the grill. It is, thus, possible for the stockboy to sneeze and for the chairman of the board to catch pneumonia from this, even though they had not seen each other. Hospital cross-infections are possible and have been reported. The same can occur in home and office buildings. Mold problems are also quite evident. Such problems should not exist if there is proper design and operation of equipment.

Physical Filtration

There are basically, among nonelectronic filters, two types of particulate filters.

1. The impaction filter depends on the dust particles striking the filter media at relatively high velocities. These are usually coated with an oil or other adhesive. National Bureau of Standards (N.B.S.) discoloration ratings for these are in the range of 5 to 10 percent removal of 1.0

micron particulate. Efficiencies are less if velocity through the filter is reduced and reentrainment of solid contaminants is a factor. These may be throw-away type or may be metal filters, i.e. washable. These have a fair dust-holding capacity. They usually emit vaporous chemical contaminants.

A. A modification of the above filter uses synthetic fibers or materials. These, with single-stage or multistage elements, are permanent and fully washable. No adhesive is added. With some of these there should be no emission of chemical contaminants and for many of this type — solid contaminants do not slough off. Efficiencies for this type tend to increase as they become "dirtier." N.B.S. discoloration efficiencies will range from 15 to 30 percent. Efficiencies do not drop off (for many of this type) with reduction of air velocities. Good dust-holding capacities exist with the multielement type.

2. The second type of filter is the diffusion filter. This filter *must* be preceded by a *good* prefilter, basically one as described in 1A. This filter is normally made of glass paper, though also available from a few sources in a non-glass media. These filters may be secured with N.B.S. discoloration ratings from 35 up through 95 percent (1.0μ contaminant removal). With the glass paper, these ratings go on up to 99.999 percent removal of 0.3 micron. These are basically white room filters as originally manufactured for the Atomic Energy Commission (A.E.C.). With adequate prefiltration, the diffusion filter will continue efficiency from one to four years. They become more efficient as they become dirty. Pressure drop depends on the velocity of air through the filter. Oversizing does not reduce efficiency and may (depending on the degree of oversizing) bring the pressure drop down to a low enough level to match residential application.

Electronic Filtration

The elctronic air cleaner or the electronic air filter that is on the market today is of the one- or two-stage type. It is stated that an electronic filter will deliver up to ten times the efficiency of the mechanical filter. (This, of course, is in comparison with the impaction filter described under 1.) The size of the contaminants removed include not only the visible dust, pollen, etc., but also contaminants down to 1.0 micron and smaller. There are certain types of contaminants that are not removed. This is frequently referred to as "white dust." The two-stage electronic air filter contains an ionization section and a collection section. Particles are first ionized and then collected on plates or other media that have the opposite charge. This is an efficient method of cleaning air; however, the ionization process and the electrical discharge between plates create an unstable form of oxygen called ozone.

The U. S. Department of Health, Education, and Welfare and the Occupational Safety and Health Administration (OSHA), as well as other health advisory and monitoring agencies, are emphatic about the necessity of not producing ozone. The problems developed by ozone on plant and animal life are theorized and clinically observed. The chemically susceptible patient quickly presents additional symptoms when exposed to ozone.

Single-stage electrostatic air purifiers clean the air without ionization of the media, at a slight reduction in initial filtration efficiency. This type of air cleaner is normally lower in cost than the two-stage.

Maintenance of any electronic air cleaner requires frequent washing of components — in many cases once or twice a week. Frequent washing of the washable components will reduce the ozone generation.

Though the electronic air cleaner removes various sizes of contaminants down through 0.1 micron and smaller, the data published indicates that the customer can expect between 85 and 90 percent N.B.S. discoloration efficiency. Some of these electronic air filters include a supplemental charcoal filter of one type or another. This charcoal filter reduces the level of household odors, reduces the ozone output, and reduces some other chemicals. Certain chemicals are *not* absorbed or reduced by the charcoal filters. Figure 11-1 presents a list that indicates what charcoal will or will not absorb.

One electronic air-cleaner manufacturer has indicated that the ozone output of their air cleaner is 0.015 parts per million. This is fifteen times stronger than the lowest value that is detectable by hypersensitive humans. It is five times stronger than the threshold of odor perception in laboratory environment with a 50 percent competence level. A concentration of 0.015 parts per million is readily detectable by most normal individuals. It has been suggested by some of the electronic air cleaner manufacturers that although they are in general agreement that the electronic air cleaner is not hazardous, the user of such equipment should be cautioned not to cloister himself in small dark rooms or any other small enclosure over prolonged periods of time with an electronic air cleaner in operation, particularly if these rooms are nearly airtight.

Technical data from one of the manufacturers of diffusion-type high efficiency filters show that the annual cost of operation of electronic air cleaners is over twice the cost of using high efficiency diffusion filters with proper prefilters.

The major question is, "Is ozone dangerous?" Many years ago, many theatres, operating rooms, infant care units, etc. had ultraviolet lamps either placed in the room or in the ducts, and air was delivered to the room via these ducts. It was soon found that some individuals became nauseated. The nausea was blamed on the ozone, which they felt was being formed by the ultraviolet lamps. Many articles have been written concerning the possible dangers of ozone. Ozone is produced by many pieces of equipment. It may come from the TV. Small amounts may come from a sewing machine motor. None, however, comes from the usual induction type of electric motor found in the home. Ozone is generated by nature during electrical storms. For an enlightening report, read "OZONE and the Electronic Air Cleaners: An Interim Report." This appeared in the trade journal *Air Conditioning, Heating and Refrigeration News*, March 9, 1970.

There are engineers who state that the ozone is not the dangerous offender, which is indicated by the following procedure: If air goes through an air duct in which there is an ozone generator, nausea may be produced; however, if, through the

Substance	Index	Substance	Index	Substance	Index
Acetaldehyde	2	Cigarette smoke odor	4	Fish odors	3
Acetic acid	4	Citrus and other fruits	4	Floral scents	4
Acetic anhydride	4	Cleaning compounds	4	Fluorotrichloromethane	3
Acetone	3	Coal smoke odor	3	Food aromas	4
Acetylene	1	Combustion odors	3	Formaldehyde	2
Acrolein	3	Cooking odors	4	Formic acid	3
Acrylic acid	4	Corrosive gases	3	Fuel gases	2
Acrylonitrile	4	Creosote	4	Fumes	3
Adhesives	4	Cresol	4	Gangrene	4
Air-Wick®	4	Crotonaldehyde	4	Garlic	4
Alcoholic beverages	4	Cyclohexane	4	Gasoline	4
Amines	2	Cyclohexanol	4	Heptane	4
Ammonia	2	Cyclohexanone	4	Heptylene	4
Amyl acetate	4	Cyclohexene	4	Hexane	3
Amyl alcohol	4	Dead animals	4	Hexylene	3
Amyl ether	4	Decane	4	Hexyne	3
Animal odors	3	Decaying substances	4	Hospital odors	4
Anesthetics	3	Deodorants	4	Household smells	4
Aniline	4	Detergents	4	Hydrogen	1
Antiseptics	4	Dibromoethane	4	Hydrogen bromide	3
Asphalt fumes	4	Dichlorobenzene	4	Hydrogen chloride	2
Automobile exhaust	3	Dichlorodifluoromethane	4	Hydrogen cyanide	3
Bathroom smells	4	Dichloroethane	4	Hydrogen fluoride	2
Benzene	4	Dichloroethylene	4	Hydrogen iodide	3
Bleaching solutions	3	Dichloroethyl ether	4	Hydrogen selenide	2
Body odors	4	Dichloromonofluormethane	3	Hydrogen sulfide	3
Borane	3	Dichloronitroethane	4	Incense	4
Bromine	4	Dichloropropane	4	Indole	4
Burned flesh	4	Dichlorotetrafluoroethane	4	Inorganic chemicals	3
Burned food	4	Diesel fumes fumeador	4	Incomplete combustion	3
Burning fat	4	Diethylamine	3	Industrial wastes	3
Butadiene	3	Diethyl ketone	4	Iodine	4
Butane	2	Dimethylaniline	4	Iodoform	4
Butanone	4	Dimethylsulfate	4	Irritants	4
Butyl acetate	4	Dioxane	4	Isophorone	4
Butyl alcohol	4	Dipropyl ketone	4	Isoprene	3
Butyl cellosolve	4	Disinfectants	4	Isophophyl acetate	4
Butyl chloride	4	Embalming odors	4	Isopropyl alcohol	4
Butyl ether	4	Ethane	1	Isopropyl ether	4
Butylene	2	Ether	3	Kerosene	4
Butyne	2	Ethyl acetate	4	Kitchen odors	4
Butyraldehyde	3	Ethyl acrylate	4	Lactic acid	4
Butyric acid	4	Ethyl alcohol	4	Lingering odors	4
Camphor	4	Ethyl amine	3	Liquid fuels	4
Cancer odor	4	Ethyl benzene	4	Liquor odors	4
Caprylic acid	4	Ethyl bromide	4	Lubricating oils and	
Carbolic acid	4	Ethyl chloride	3	greases	4
Carbon disulfide	4	Ethyl ether	3	Lysol®	4
Carbon dioxide	1	Ethyl formate	3	Masking agents	4
Carbon monoxide	1	Ethyl mercaptan	3	Medicinal odors	4
Carbon tetrachloride	4	Ethyl silicate	4	Melons	4
Cellosolve®	4	Ethylene	1	Menthol	4
Cellosolve® acetate	4	Ethylene chlorhydrin	4	Mercaptans	4
Charred materials	4	Ethylene dichloride	4	Mesityl oxide	4
Cheese	4	Ethylene oxide	3	Methane	1
Chlorine	3	Essential oils	4	Methyl acetate	3
Chlorobenzene	4	Eucalyptole	4	Methyl acrylate	4
Chlorobutadiene	4	Exhaust fumes	3	Methyl alcohol	3
Chloroform	4	Female odors	4	Methyl bromide	3
Chloronitropropane	4	Fertilizer	4	Methyl butyl ketone	4
Chloropicrin®	4	Film Processing odors	3	Methyl cellosolve®	4

Figure 11-1. Chemical fumes adsorption by activated charcoal.

Substance	Index	Substance	Index	Substance	Index
Methyl cellosolve® acetate	4	Palmitic acid	4	Sewer odors	4
Methyl chloride	3	Paper deteriorations	4	Skatole	4
Methyl Chloroform	4	Paradichlorbenzine	4	Slaughtering odors	3
Methyl ether	3	Paste and glue	4	Smog	4
Methyl ethyl ketone	4	Pentane	3	Soaps	4
Methyl formate	3	Pentanone	4	Smoke	4
Methyl isobutyl ketone	4	Pentylene	3	Solvents	3
Methyl mercaptan	4	Pentyne	3	Sour milks	4
Methylcyclohexane	4	Perchloroethylene	4	Spilled beverages	4
Methycyclohexanol	4	Perfumes, cosmetics	4	Spoiled food stuffs	4
Methycyclohexanone	4	Perspirations	4	Stale odors	4
Methylene chloride	4	Persistent odors	4	Stoddard solvent	4
Mildew	3	Pet odors	4	Stuffiness	4
Mixed odors	4	Phenol	4	Styrene monomer	4
Mold	3	Phosgene	3	Sulfur dioxide	2
Monochlorobenzene	4	Pitch	4	Sulfur trioxide	3
Monofluorotri-		Plastics	4	Sulfuric acid	4
chloromethane	4	Poison gases	3	Tar	4
Moth balls	4	Pollen	3	Tarnishing gases	3
Naphtha (coal tar)	4	Popcorn and candy	4	Tetrachloroethane	4
Naphtha (petroleum)	4	Poultry odors	4	Tetrachloroethylene	4
Naphthalene	4	Propane	2	Theatrical makeup odors	4
Nicotine	4	Propionaldehyde	3	Tobacco smoke odor	4
Nitric acid	3	Propionic acid	4	Toilet odors	4
Nitro benzenes	4	Propyl acetate	4	Toluene	4
Nitroethane	4	Propyl alcohol	4	Toluidine	4
Nitrogen dioxide	2	Propyl chloride	4	Trichlorethylene	4
Nitroglycerine	4	Propyl ether	4	Trichloroethane	4
Nitromethane	4	Propyl Mercaptan	4	Turpentine	4
Nitropropane	4	Propylene	2	Urea	4
Nitrotoluene	4	Propyne	2	Uric acid	4
Nonane	4	Putrefying substances	3	Valeric acid	4
Noxious gases	3	Putrescine	4	Valericaldehyde	4
Octalene	4	Pyridine	4	Varnish fumes	4
Octane	4	Radiation products	2	Vinegar	4
Odorants	4	Rancid oils	4	Vinyl chloride	3
Onions	4	Resins	4	Volatile materials	3
Organic chemicals	4	Reodorants	4	Waste products	4
Ozone	4	Ripening fruits	4	Wood alcohol	3
Packing house odors	4	Rubber	4	Xylene	4
Paint & Redecorating odors	4	Sauerkraut	4		

Some of the contaminants listed in the table are specific chemical compounds, some represent classes of compounds, and others are mixtures and of variable composition. Activated charcoal's capacity for odors varies somewhat with the concentration in air, with humidity and temperature, and with the actual velocity used through the filters. The numbers given represent typical or average conditions and might vary in specific instances. The values in the table have been assembled from many sources including laboratory tests and field experience. In cases where numerical values were not available, the author has listed his opinion of the probable capacity based on general experience. The table should be used as a general rule only.

The capacity index has the following meaning:—

4. High capacity for all materials in this category. One pound takes up about 20% to 50% of its own weight—average about 1/3 (33 1/3%). This category includes most of the odor causing substances.

3. Satisfactory capacity for all items in this category. These constitute good applications but the capacity is not as high as for category 4. Absorbs about 10 to 25% of its weight—average about 1/6 (16.7%).

2. Includes substances which are not highly adsorbed but which might be taken up sufficiently to give good service under the particular conditions of operation. These require individual checking.

1. Adsorption capacity is low for these materials. Activated charcoal cannot be satisfactorily used to remove them under ordinary circumstances.

same duct with an ozone generator, pure oxygen is transmitted, no nausea is observed by breathing the effluent from the duct. This may be attributed to the fact that there is nitrogen, sulphur, and other chemicals in the air that are oxidized by the ozone. Oxides of these compounds are known to be harmful. This enhances my thinking in the basic premise that we must do as much as possible *not* to produce oxidized pollutants. Thus, it is believed by many that ozone is not in itself a dangerous material, but that because of its instability, it combines with sulphur, nitrogen and possibly other elements to form compounds that are dangerous to all living forms and particularly to the chemically susceptible individual.

If the electronic air cleaner can produce ozone and if ozone is capable of producing dangerous compounds, how can we advocate the use of this type of filtration unless we follow this filter with some type of suitable chemical filtration?

Chemical Filtration

The suitable filtration unit may be one of several types. It may be placed in the ductwork of the air conditioning unit or of the warm-air furnace. It may be a portable unit that sits anyplace in the room — in any room. It may be a filter built into the wall of each room that filters the air coming from the outside into the inside. The type of filter that we have found to be relatively safe (whatever air cleaning may be used, someone may be sensitive to it) is as follows:

It has been found that many patients are hypersensitive to potassium permanganate. A combination of the potassium permanganate with other materials usually answers the problems in most of these cases. Charcoal filters may produce discomforting reaction in some individuals. This problem can be overcome. For the hypersensitive individual, or should I say the ultrahypersensitive individual, it may take additional research to find the right combination of materials for air filtration to meet a specific individual's requirements.

It has been established that most individuals can tolerate nonelectronic filters set up in the following manner:

1. A prefilter of multistage construction that includes a coarse screen of metal or synthetic material followed by medium synthetic nonwoven fabric and followed by a nylon or Dacron® dense nonwoven fabric. All of this is in a permanent metal frame. This is washable in a biodegradable cleaning material at one- to two-month intervals.
2. A combination of coconut shell activated charcoal filters and *Purafil®* filters, in proper order and with necessary seals, to remove the various gaseous chemical contaminants.
3. A high efficiency particulate filter to remove (normally) 95 percent of 1.0 micron material, 55 percent of 0.3 micron particulate.

The order of the components can be critical.

A sniff test of the various components of every filter unit by the patient may indicate whether problems exist. For physicians who have filtration units in their offices, the patient can be placed in close proximity to the unit and instructed to breathe the air directly from the unit. After several minutes, this will determine the existence of compatability. Also, the patient can secure a unit on rental for prolonged testing and evaluation. Still another possibility is a small test unit from which the patient can breathe the air for an extended period.

In summary, the removal of particulate matter from the indoor atmosphere is accomplished by suitable filtration. Which method is used depends upon which is acceptable to the individual.

Chapter 12

ECOLOGY OF HOUSEHOLD SUPPLIES

Francis Silver

SELECTION of janitorial and household supplies is a matter of great importance if the air in buildings is to be maintained in a condition conducive to health. Seldom today is much thought given to such problems. What we see emphasized instead of health are esthetics, convenience, or cheap price. An intense, competitive sales pressure prevails for a wide variety of products whose use, as recommended, will seriously contaminate the indoor air. The sales pressure is applied to housekeepers, janitors, and others who are poorly prepared to assess the health consequences of their selections.

Parallel with the trend to use chemical remedies for as many agricultural problems as possible, there has been the growing tendency to offer chemicals for an increasing number of household problems. The producers of household supplies sponsor massive public relations programs that overshadow the undesirable side effects of such chemicals. As a consequence of such massive promotion, it is hardly an exaggeration to state, for instance, that more unintentional prescribing is done by service personnel in hospitals than intentional prescribing by physicians. Probably the chief competitors to the physicians' medications are the exterminators with their sprays and fumigations. The painters with their outgassing petrochemical paints are overwhelming in this respect. And the janitors and housekeeping maids with their aromatic and phenolic sanitizing chemicals are the more persistent polluters of the indoor environment.

What has been said about the hospital situation is similarly true of the domestic environment. The homemaker determines the intake of chemicals by the members of the family on a daily basis; whereas, the physician prescribes only occasionally. Some studies also indicate that inhaled chemicals can negate the physicians' treatments. This problem of pollution by household supplies has evoked an informal proposal by the government to classify paints for indoor use as a prescription item.

It has long been known in informed circles that, if a product which will evaporate is sprayed into the air or spread over a large surface inside a building, a substantial portion of that product will end up inside the occupants of that building. This occurs because of the large volume of air required for breathing (several thousand gallons of air is inhaled daily by every individual) and the efficient absorptive capability of the lungs.

Skin absorption also might be significant for many compounds released into the air because of the many square feet of exposed body tissue. Because of the numerous synthetic materials of clothing, bedding, and furniture, the direct contact exposure is long and intimate. Chemical formula changes of synthetics and new treatments of natural and synthetic products, such as fire retardants and antistatic agents, might be adverse to the chemically susceptible individual.

To emphasize the hazards of inhaled chemicals, the use or storage of any toxic substance inside an inhabited building should be kept to a minimum. When toxic chemicals must be used inside inhabited buildings, we should select those products which will be of such extremely low volatility that the fumes from them will be highly diluted by the inhaled air. Spraying any product into the air indoors should be strictly avoided as a routine practice. When products such as paints, cleaners, or disinfectants, which do evaporate severely, must be used indoors, they should be applied by personnel who wear protective masks. Also, adequate time should be allowed for ventilation and complete evaporation after the chemicals are applied to assure removal from the indoor air of residual contaminants. In buildings where forced air systems comingle the atmosphere from various rooms, it may be necessary to close the forced air registers to a specific room that is being treated and utilize windows for its ventilation. The architectural trend toward sealed structures will make some of these recommended precautions impossible. Alternate means of purging the contaminated air should be developed.

The environmental rule to keep the use and storage of volatile toxic substances outside the living or the work space to a maximum is not new. We were taught this in gas engineering courses at Johns Hopkins University prior to 1937. Complying with this rule leaves any chemical substance subject to question, except pure water and inert chemicals. The reasons for honoring this rule are two-fold: (1) the need of avoiding chemical sensitization, and (2) the need of avoiding slow (chronic) poisoning. Although both of these points are well understood in informed circles and they are adequately proven with extensive documentation, there still exists a substantially strong public indifference to such hazards.

The scientifically established reasoning on which the second point in the preceding discussion rests is illustrated by the following bit of medical history: Quicksilver (mercury) had long been used in quantities of one to two pounds per dose to be taken by mouth for intestinal obstruction prior to 1900 A.D. Although some persons are sensitive to mercury and may have been sickened or killed by this heroic approach, it is believed that some patients were saved by the use of mercury for medication of abdominal obstruction. If the same amount of mercury, which most individuals could drink with little effect, is spilled on the floor in a confined room and the fumes arising are inhaled over a prolonged period of time, chronic poisoning results therefrom. The oral mercury caused only a moderate amount of trouble because its low water solubility prevented its absorption, and it was soon eliminated from the body.

The extremely rapid and copious absorption through the lungs is another story. Chronic mercury poisoning by inhalation is so well known as to have earned a place in the medical dictionary. It is defined as *erythismus mercurialis*, which is a psychical disturbance noted in persons poisoned with mercury. It is characterized by timidity, especially in the presence of strangers (1). The characterisitics of the psychical disturbances by chronic poisoning from mercury have been enshrined in the literature of the Mad Hatter and by *Alice in Wonderland*. Chronic mercury poisoning was an occupational disease in the hat industry until recently. The Mad Hatter trembled and shook when the Queen of Hearts pointed her finger at him.

Tremor and fearfulness were characteristic of this disease.

Probably the worst items in American homes are the moth-killing chemicals — namely, paradichlorobenzene and naphthalene. They come in the form of moth crystals, nuggets, cakes, balls, and flakes. These chemicals I would estimate to produce more injury than is produced by automobile accidents. None of these products should ever be used in the home. Their use as recommended has produced headaches, high blood pressure, cataracts, liver and kidney disturbance, in addition to damaging the complexion of many individuals. Moth treatment should be dealt with by mechanical means, such as covering garments with plastic bags, sunning, airing, and brushing them. Moths and their eggs are fragile and cannot endure activity. Moths cannot live in a blanket on the bed you sleep in, nor in a suit you wear once a week, even if the suit hangs in a moth-infested closet the remainder of the week. Several articles have been written about harmless ways for dealing with moths (2,3).

Currently a disinfectant spray, yellow insecticide strips, and aerosol dispensers are vying with each other to see which will become the most health-damaging item in the American home. Despite the widespread promotion, it is doubtful if any of these items should ever be used in the home. There are safer remedies for all of the problems with which they propose to deal. The dangerous lindane and the DDT in a vaporizer have been replaced by the yellow strip and by the timed-mist dispenser, which are also harmful to human health.

Chemically harmless cleaning methods have been amply demonstrated. Doctor Lawrence Dickey, in the ecology ward of his hospital, required the housekeeping personnel to scrub floors with a borax solution. The solution consisted of one-half cup of borax to one gallon of hot water. After monitoring this procedure for a period of one year by a bacteriologist it was reported that the borax solution satisfied germicidal requirements. The bacterial colony count was as low in the area where borax solution was used as in the remainder of the hospital where aromatic chemicals were used.

In general, old-fashioned mineral-type products used by our mothers and grandmothers are of lower volatility and, hence, safer as far as air purity is concerned. Reference here is to such items as baking soda, washing soda, borax, trisodium phosphate, Oakite®, and lye.

Baking soda makes an excellent cleanser for sanitizing food storage refrigerators. Its low toxicity is demonstrated when one-half teaspoon in a glassful of water is used for a sour stomach.

Washing soda is strongly alkaline and should be used with care. It is almost as good a bleach as chlorine compounds, but it does not emit fumes, nor does it rot the clothes.

Oakite was long the preferred substance for washing painted walls. Unfortunately, it is hard to find in the stores presently.

Chlorine and ammonia give off fumes, but these fumes dissipate quickly. Occasional use might be acceptable, provided their hazard is understood and the sensitive individuals are protected from exposure to such fumes. Because fumes from chlorine and ammonia dissipate so quickly, they usually cause less trouble than standard insecticides. They may be used instead of PCB or PBB and other such chemicals.

The newer, volatile cleaning agents are to be avoided. They give off fumes for a long time after they are used on floors and walls. The same disadvantages characterize rug cleaners and are one of the factors that help make fastened-down carpet inadvisable.

Some of the linoleum coverings do not require waxing. Although such covering is usually put down with an asphalt glue that can give off some fumes for a time, it soon loses that effect and provides an excellent floor finish. Similar comments apply to polyurethane varnish over hardwood floors. Although varnish is extremely toxic while drying, it usually outgasses in a few days and does not require waxing thereafter. Modern varnishes are much more durable than older varnishes. There are three types of varnish — high gloss; satin finish, which is a medium gloss; and low gloss, which is reported not to hold up well. In contemplation of using varnish, the chemically susceptible individual should be tested for tolerance to a given brand of varnish with the painted-board technique.

Homemakers should form the habit of wearing rubber gloves for scrubbing or for washing dishes. This will protect the hands from toxic detergents, which are activated frequently by the warmth of the water. In this connection I recall that when I entered Johns Hopkins University in 1934, a classmate was having trouble with his hands. His family had a restaurant, and the strong soap to which he was exposed caused skin trouble. More recently, a friend took over her parents' restaurant. In just a few years, her hands resembled those of my classmate during my undergraduate years. I strongly recommended to her that she obtain rubber gloves and use them during dishwashing. She discovered that in addition to protection against the detergent, she could increase the water temperature without increasing discomfort from the heat. Care should be taken, however, in selecting rubber gloves so that they do not add to the chemical problem of the detergent. Generally, rubber gloves emitting a strong odor when immersed in hot water should be suspected of probable toxic effect.

It should be stated here that some mild liquid detergents are tolerable if exposure to them is infrequent. For daily use as dishwashing additives, protective gloves are recommended, especially for the hypersensitive individual.

If floor waxing is deemed necessary, then the hard paste waxes are to be preferred instead of the liquid waxes. Hard paste waxes ordinarily will only need to be applied once or twice a year because of their greater durability. The waxing should be done in warm weather so that the fumes the wax produces, which are chiefly turpentine, can be aired during application and after application for several days. Once the application and fumigation is completed, several months of freedom from fumes prevails. The softer waxes and liquid waxes, which claim to be self-polishing, require frequent application, and they tend to outgas heavily. With weekly, or more frequent, application of these waxes, the atmosphere in the room tends to linger, which enhances the aggravation for the chemically susceptible individual.

For furniture polishing the hard paste waxes are much to be preferred instead of the usual liquid polishes. Although more effort is required for the first application of a hard paste wax to furniture, it should last several years per application, and it will be less troublesome from the outgassing on the overall period. Between the infrequent waxing, dusting with a felt cloth should be sufficient. The vacuum cleaner can be used to lift the dust as an alternate method of cleaning waxed furniture. Frequent smearing of the furniture with products purported to remove dust, which are volatile and smell of aromatic oil, cannot be done without having a probable health hazard. For chemically susceptible persons such exposures will often prove incapacitating. For the acutely sensitive individuals, it may be necessary to refrain from any waxes, polishes, or cleaners. In such situations a damp-cloth treatment may be the only solution.

Silver- and brass-polishing chemicals are generally toxic. Salt and vinegar mixed together makes a safer cleaner for such metals as silver, brass, and copper. Silverware can be cleaned by putting it in an aluminum pan that is filled with hot water and that has cream of tartar or baking soda added to it. This method requires less effort and seemingly does not harm the silver. If the commercial silver polish must be used, it should only be used outdoors, and the user should refrain from inhaling the fumes emitted by the cleaning chemical.

Aromatic disinfectants should never be used in the home. The current advertising that suggests that everything in the house should be sprayed frequently with materials which contain carbolic acid or diphenyl is dangerous and expensive advice. In my consultation work I occasionally encounter a household where odorous chemicals are utilized for sanitizing purposes. The results are uniformly adverse with reference to mental, as well as physical, disturbance. In one situation of my acquaintance, it has taken more than a year of heavy cross ventilation to completely eliminate the unhealthful effect of one spraying of two and one-half ounces of a widely promoted disinfectant solution.

For window cleaning a solution of one cup of vinegar in a gallon of hot water is preferred. Ammonia solution is an alternate window cleanser, and some of the spray-type cleaners are least desirable for individuals with chemical susceptibility. To eliminate direct contact with the chemicals of window cleaners, the solution should be applied with a long-handled brush, and the window should be dried with a squeegee.

Room deodorizers should be particularly avoided because

they tend to distort the sense of smell. Furthermore, these chemicals are toxic and incite discomforting symptoms in chemically susceptible individuals. Most importantly, however, the damaging of the sense of smell destroys our ability to detect spoiled food, smoldering electrical fires, and other odoriferous hazards.

Organic insecticides, which have been introduced since World War II, and which contain such substances as DDT, chlordane, malathion, diazinon, etc., must not be used indoors, or the facility may be permanently contaminated and become intolerable to a sensitive person. Much safer substances are available for use in occupied buildings, such as sodium fluoride, borax, or boric acid. Such minerals can be added to an attractive bait made of powdered sugar, flour and cocoa. From 10 to 50 percent concentration will provide adequate toxicity for household insects (4,5).

Ralph Doty in *Mother Earth News*, number 43 on page 143, recommends baking soda to kill roaches. The baking soda gives off carbon dioxide gas in reaction with the stomach acids, and since the roaches are unable to belch, this kills them. To make the baking soda more attractive to the roaches, mix it with some powdered sugar.

Since reading about the use of baking soda for roach extermination, several persons have told me that baking soda is a very old and highly effective roach treatment. Actually, baking soda is superior to the commonly used sodium flouride and has less poisonous hazard for humans. During World War II the navy ships used a mixture of one part flour to one part plaster of paris for roach control. This method proved to be unusually effective. With these proven old remedies that are available to everyone, there is no need to use the newer, but more toxic, organic pesticides.

It is not commonly recognized that dye coloring is hazardous to the chemically susceptible individual. The health of many persons has been jeopardized by hair dyes and hair tints. Eye shadow has had an unsavory record of eye damage. It is unrealistic to expect government protection from such chemical exposures. Furthermore, the problem of chemical susceptibility is too new to expect existing laws to cover all recent developments. For example, little is known about the effect of perfume on human health, but it has been established that aromatic hydrocarbons are harmful to human health. One of the simplest aromatic compounds, benzene, which gives the sweet and pleasant odor to rubber cement, was early established as a cause of leukemia (6,7). Dyes derived from hydrocarbons should be avoided. Garments that come in direct contact with the skin should be free of heavy and dark coloring. Paper goods, such as facial tissue and toilet tissue, that come in contact with the moist and delicate skin tissues should be free of unstable coloring.

Selecting laundry detergents is a matter of trial and error. What one can tolerate, another may find to be highly offensive. Basically, if you have found something satisfactory, do not try other unproven products just to save a few pennies on the purchase price.

Some enzymes have been found to be troublesome. The detergents that are represented as having a violent action in getting the dirt out should probably be avoided in favor of something more gentle. Cosmetics also should be as simple as possible. Do not take chances testing sample products, you are under no obligation to try out the sample sent to you simply because it is a free gift.

More details regarding the changes in control of the chemical environment within the home will be found elsewhere in this book. There has been a major loss of environmental control since World War II. This makes it imperative for today's homemaker to become fully informed about the health hazards related to the use of any domestic product.

The future is certainly not encouraging. There seems little likelihood of overall improvement coming from any major source to the householder. Every obnoxious product that is taken off the market is quickly replaced by two or three items with a worse effect on human health. Although the government has been reasonably effective in curbing general ambient pollution from sulfur dioxide, its action in regard to health hazards from household chemicals is too insignificant for reassurance of a brighter future. Consequently, each homemaker will be well advised to monitor carefully all household supplies intended for use in the family's home.

BIBLIOGRAPHY

1. Dorland, W.A.N.: *The American Illustrated Medical Dictionary*, 21st ed. Philadelphia, Saunders, 1948, p. 514.
2. Silver, F.: Practical Insect Control. *Natural Food and Farming*, Jan. 1965, pp. 27-34.
3. Silver, F: Insect control. In Golos, N. (Ed.): *Management of Complex Allergies*. Norwalk, Conn., New England Foundation for Allergic and Environmental Disease, pp. 124-134. Available from New England Foundation for Allergic and Environmental Disease, 3 Bush Street, Norwalk, Connecticut 06850.
4. Silver, F.: letter regarding problems created by using chlordane in the home. In Pottenger, F.M., Jr.: *Proceedings — The National Conference on Water Pollution*. Washington, D.C., December 12-14, 1960.
5. Petty, C.S.: Case histories from work carried on at the Louisiana State University School of Medicine 1955 to 1958 under U. S. Army Chemical Corps Contract No. DA 18-108-CML5473, appendix 5 of the report. Malathion stored in an office caused marked psychic changes. Proven by tests.
6. Stabile, Toni: Nobody calls it dye anymore. *Cosmetics, Trick or Treat*. New York, Hawthorn, 1966, pp. 126-137.
7. Salter, Wm. T.: Benzene & leukemia. *A Textbook of Pharmacology*. Philadelphia, Saunders, 1952, pp. 936-937.
8. Silver, F.: The plastic problem in environmental engineering. *The Human Ecology Study Group Feb. 1976 Newsletter*, pp. 7, 8; *Spring Newsletter*, p. 4, 5.
9. *Ecologist*, Feb. 1976, pp. 2-4, May 1976, p. 9.

Chapter 13

WATER ECOLOGY FOR HYPERSENSITIVES

Casimir M. Nikel

FOR the purpose of this chapter the term *hypersensitive* will mean a person who experiences an undesirable reaction from water, regardless of the water makeup, except for the bacterial and viral content of the water. Reaction to the latter, of course, is known as an infection.

Research of water ecology has revealed that its complexity is too much for one monograph. Books from such eminent authors as Andrews, Carson, and Deming prove this contention. Water is not only the ultimate life-support system, but it is almost impossible to obtain it in a pure form. One might therefore ask, "How can we escape the consequences of contaminated water? In fact, is there such a thing as an unfavorable reaction to water?" Discussion under separate subheadings may cast some enlightening information on the subject.

WATER FOR LIFE SUPPORT

If a street survey were to ask, "Without which single substance would life perish?" the answer would probably be, "Air." This probably would be derived from personal experience. We generally accept the view that five minutes without the oxygen in the air would result in certain death. Yet, it has been proven that anaerobic organisms can live without oxygen.

Experience also teaches that a human can lose 50 percent of body protein and almost all of the body fat and still survive (1). In the case of prolonged fasts, such as abstinence from food for forty days, most persons will survive the rigorous experience. However, 10 percent loss of our body water content can mean certain death.

Water seems to be the ultimate life-support substance. Scientists are convinced that all life must have water. If traces of water could have been found on Mars this would have been positive proof to the scientists that life might exist there.

It is thought that human life originated in primitive oceans. One reason for this belief is that when ocean water is diluted with distilled water on a one to twenty ratio, it has almost the exact salty makeup as human blood.

If the human body has a 1 percent decrease in the normal water content, a sensation of thirst develops. Hunger and suffocation require at least seven times more decrease of air or food before these sensations occur, which suggests the importance of water.

The human body almost floats in water. Sixty to seventy-five percent of our body consists of water. An average 150-pound man would produce approximately 108 pounds of water if he were squeezed like a sponge in a giant hand. That amounts to nine gallons of water in an average-sized man. How then can an individual be hypersensitive to water?

Morgan in his study found at least a dozen symptoms of major illness from water (2). These findings included everything from a runny nose, to asthma, to disturbance of the nervous system. Presumably this is due to chemical susceptibility. The orthomolecular effect may also have something to do with hypersensitivity to water (3).

CHEMISTRY OF WATER

The chemistry of water could be considered as rather simple. Water contains only two elements. Both of them are abundant in nature. They are hydrogen and oxygen (H_2O). These elements, when combined on a two to one ratio, result in a silky soft liquid that flows, evaporates into the atmosphere, condenses into fog or cloud formation, and, under proper thermal conditions, falls back to earth in the form of raindrops or hailstones.

When water falls upon the earth, most of it soaks into the ground. Some of it runs off and finds gulleys that connect to streams and rivers, all leading downgrade toward lakes, seas, and oceans. But, an important portion of this water is that which the earth absorbs and forms into aquifers (4). These aquifers consist of underground rivers and lakes — some go to a depth of 1,500 to 2,500 feet below the surface of the topsoil. This accumulation of underground waters makes possible a multibillion dollar, agriculturally-related industry in such arid places as Palestine, the southwestern United States, Mexico, and elsewhere. All of this indicates what an important single substance for life support water seems to be.

The process of evaporation, rainfall, and ground absorption complicates the chemistry of water. Because water is such an effective solvent, it accumulates various dissolved solids and gases in its travel from the ocean into the atmosphere and down into the earth from where we extract it through springs and wells.

Under chemical analysis water becomes more than just H_2O. As a result of aeration, water accumulates free-floating oxygen. This makes underwater life of fish and plants possible. Curiously, when an overabundance of organic life develops, it robs the water of free-floating oxygen, and the fish suffocate.

The prevailing solvent quality of water dissolves free hydrogen into it as it dissolves various compounds in the soil. This changes its pH, which is a measure of acidity. At a pH of 7, water is considered chemically neutral, which is within the pH range of the human blood and biological cells.

As a result of the reactions with compounds and the input from decaying plant life, the water becomes sufficiently acidic to be corrosive. A recent United States Public Health Service report stated that "water having a pH of 6 or lower should be strongly suspected of contamination and should not be used until confirmed otherwise." In view of the foregoing warning, it is distressing to note that Pfeiffer reports water supplies that have a pH level of 4 and lower are regularly consumed, which has resulted in a tragic infant death in one situation.

It might be assumed that the pH value of water reacts indirectly on a hypersensitive individual in its more acidic state, particularly since acids are known to be powerful oxidizers. In this state water tends to dissolve heavy metals. The dissolved heavy metals float in the water as invisible ions.

Heavy metals are known to be toxic to the human body. It

could be presumed that when water contaminated with heavy metals is ingested, these contaminants could react against the human cells in various parts of the body. This might be a sort of transcellular effect that some medical authorities identify as allergic reactions. Hence, an individual with chemical susceptibility might react to ingested water.

Some of the chemicals* that water dissolves give water a quality termed hardness. The principal chemicals resulting in water hardness are calcium, magnesium, and iron. In ionic form these chemicals tend to produce flocculations in reaction with other chemicals that are contained, for example, in common household soap. The flocculations interfere with laundering, bathing, and various industrial processes. Such chemical reactions suggest what might be happening inside the human body when the various ionic chemical elements are ingested with water. Recent scientific investigations confirm this suspicion (12,13).

It is definite that water is not only a complex chemical substance, but it also possesses various harmful physical characteristics. Ecologists test water for approximately a dozen major characteristics. These consist of such factors as dissolved particles and gas content, hardness, pH value, turbidity, temperature, etc. The last of these characteristics is extremely important, especially for fish life. Most fish can tolerate water temperatures between 35°F and a top level of 75°F.

Chemists know that chemical reactions can be accelerated by increase of temperature. This might have something to do with hypersensitivity, since the human body maintains a temperature in excess of 98°F. This might also suggest why a hypersensitive individual reacts to water from one water spring source, but not from another, since different chemicals react at different temperature levels. Even rain water, which is generally considered as least contaminated, "contains carbon dioxide, chloride, sulfates, nitrates and ammonia, with organic and inorganic dust" (6). We are told that "all water that flows over the earth contains inorganic and organic dissolved and sus-

---

*"Chemical" in this setting is used in the broad sense, referring to dissolved solids as well as gaseous substances.

pended matter" (7). Some authorities report that man-made chemicals (many of them highly toxic) are to be found in all waters, not only in streams at the top of the highest mountains, but also in most of the underground water.

From this it can be seen that water chemistry is highly complex. Some of its chemical complexity is the result of man-made pollution. Probably the most dramatic presentation of the universal pollution of water is Rachel Carson's *Silent Spring*. However, since Carson's alert to the water problem, sufficient number of reliable scientists have joined the ranks in support of Carson's position that no apology or justification is necessary to claim that water chemistry is not only complex, but it is also hazardous to the human organism. Water is especially hazardous to a human afflicted with hypersensitivity.

ECOLOGY OF WATER

Ecologists are beginning to study water as assiduously as the chemists have done since empirical science started serious investigation of water's molecular structure (by John Dalton in 1808). Some very curious phenomena suggest that water ecology involves physical factors as well as chemical factors. Chemically water is very stable. For instance, the atomic bond between water's oxygen and hydrogen remains intact although water is heated to 1,000°C. On the other hand, water's physical form changes to a vapor at 100°C.

Ecologists find that water life forms are greatly affected by the associated physical elements of water. For instance, water at 35°F supports a different fish than water at 75°F. Interestingly, even movement of water seems to produce an ecologic effect. Trout prefer a cool mountain stream, while pike prefer cool lake water, which is less turbulent.

Water scientists are beginning to ask such questions as, "Why are leeches found in sluggish streams? Why do mosquitoes breed in stagnant waters? Why do crayfish prefer streams with rocky bottoms? In what ways do water characteristics affect living organisms?" (9).

What seems to be true of water ecology in reference to wildlife seems similarly true of water ecology in reference to human beings. This is suggested by Morgan's study referred to previously. Andrews, et al. state that "it is not enough to study man alone, water alone, or plants alone. The study must relate to all living things and to their environments" (10). Since "all water that flows over the earth . . . contains inorganic and organic dissolved and suspended matter," physicians practicing clinical ecology find it increasingly important to consider water ecology in the treatment of patients (7).

WATER POLLUTION, PIPING, AND PURIFICATION

In the study of water ecology, not all substances contained in liquid water* can be considered as pollution. "The natural nutrients in waters are nature's way of polluting her waters" according to Andrews, et al. (11). How can a pollutant be a nutrient? Or why should someting nutritious be considered as a pollutant? Substances in water are only pollutants in the context of this chapter if they are harmful to human beings. Their presence may actually be needed by water organisms, water plants, fish, or other mammals than humans.

In the earlier history of water treatment for its use by human beings removal of suspended solids seemed most important. When large cities developed, engineering scientists gathered water into large pools for sedimentation purposes. Historically, this was the first stage of purification in an attempt to provide large amounts of potable water. Later, a method of percolating water through sand developed in an attempt to arrive at a greater degree of purification. Probably the greatest advance in developing potable water came with the use of chlorine. This chemical was found to have the capability of killing the hardiest bacteria known to man, until recently. Chlorine, in the concentrations and time of contact currently used in water treatment, does not satisfactorily kill virus. Long storage aeration and ultraviolet lights are being considered alternate water-treating techniques.

The most recent experience with potable water has revealed

---

*Water is found in three physical forms — solid, in ice form; gaseous, in vapor or steam form; and liquid, the most familiar form.

to clinical ecologists that many patients react to ordinary water. Clinical observation indicates that not all hypersensitives, however, react alike to the same water. In fact, the same patient does not react the same to waters from various sources. Some recent reports indicate that some hypersensitives react to water that has been distilled. A most puzzling observation has been temporary tolerance for water from a given source with intolerance developing after extended use.

Reaction to distilled water poses some probable explanations. Since water is a potent solvent, at high temperatures it might erode the structure of the still and bring chemicals in molecular and ionized form to the user of distilled water. Pfeiffer reports that water with a low pH erodes copper piping so that pinholes develop in ten years after installation of house plumbing (14). It has been established that despite trace amount needs in the human body for copper, excess amounts are toxic. If such a heavy and hard metal as copper in plumbing is dissolved by water at ambient temperature, then it may react chemically and physically more so at the higher temperatures during distillation. This could result in a transport of heavy metals to a hypersensitive person and conceivably could result in a biochemical reaction.

This problem with distilled water is well established in the medical profession. The manufacturers in the health industry have tried to overcome the water ecology difficulties by building stills from glass. In spite of such heroic efforts, pyrogenic infections and physiological disturbances in patients persisted. During the 1950s I visited Johns Hopkins University Hospital and discussed the problem of pyrogenics with some of the medical personnel there. Some of them speculated that nonglass connectors may have been responsible. Presumably this was changed, but as far as present information is available to me, the problem of pyrogenics is still with us.

If a hypersensitive person was to request a recommendation for a source of totally safe water, I would have no absolute suggestion. The chemical pollutions from factories, farms, service institutions, and domestic sources make all potable waters suspect (13). Although half a dozen methods for water purification exist, none can produce water that is totally free of some substance which might disturb a hypersensitive individual.

Early in the history of our country conventional plumbing consisted of lead and galvanized piping. It was discovered that water leached the lead in the piping, so copper became a universal substitute. However, the joining of copper pipes still uses solder, which is a lead-containing metal. Water at a low pH level dissolves copper and lead. Consequently many of the chronic illnesses may actually be a low-level poisoning by heavy metals ingested with potable water (12). Although the federal government attempts to protect us through the Environmental Protection Agency, the implementation of legislation and coordination of scientific and medical findings is slow. In view of such discrepancies, a hypersensitive individual should suspect all approved sources of water.

An unprofessional approach to meet water ecology problems by a hypersensitive individual suggests several steps:

1. Use water only from a known source. (Its quality should at least meet the requirements of the United States Public Health Service drinking water standards.)

2. Boiling potable water may render it more tolerable to a hypersensitive individual. (In view of recent chlorine-related carcinogenic findings, it might be advisable for everybody to boil potable water from a public utility source.)

3. Filtration of potable water through an activated charcoal cell might be helpful. (Many hardware stores sell these for as little as thirty dollars per unit. The original unit is renewable with an inexpensive disposable cartridge.)

4. Use of deionized water, which is available in most supermarkets, is a convenient alternate source. (Be sure that this water comes in glass containers. Plastic should be absolutely avoided by the hypersensitive person.)

5. Finally, distillation might be considered as a potential source of potable water. Distillation, however, is not a complete assurance of water purity. One authority states that "distilling units are often represented as the ideal way to purify water. With proper precautions, distillation separates water from non-volatile components such as salt or lime. The story with volatile components, however, is

very different. Based on Dalton's law of partial pressures and steam distillation, this process is a poor method for separating water from volatile chemicals. Such chemicals as the modern pesticides, chlorine, or ammonia will carry-over with the water into the final distillate" (16).

It has been reported that even triple distillation has proven insufficient to produce tolerable water for some hypersensitive patients. In such circumstances it is suggested that the distilled water be boiled in an open kettle for at least twenty minutes. The boiling kettle should be made of glass or stainless steel to minimize contamination.

In summary, one must recognize that no ultimate conclusions are available from the present state of the art. Clinical ecologists are probably the most expert in helping a hypersensitive individual understand his problem with water ecology.

Too often we may be misled by assuming that it is what goes in the mouth that defiles a person (15). Actually, it may be the chemistry of the individual that reacts to a reasonably good and acceptable water. During my many years in a hospital situation, I have seen such patients. They were too ill to tolerate water, even in teaspoon quantities. In such cases the physician infused the water intravenously until such time that the patient could tolerate a normal intake.

In the case of a hypersensitive individual, he may be mobile, but his insides may be too sick to tolerate water from usual sources. The illness could be of such a nature as not to be correctable by mere passage of time. In such circumstances the person ought to seek out a physician who is acquainted with clinical ecology and submit to such a physician's ministrations.

BIBLIOGRAPHY

1. Deming, H.G.: *Water: The Fountain of Opportunity*. Fair Lawn, New Jersey, Ox U Pr, 1975, pp. 145-147.
2. Morgan, Joseph T.: The water problem. In Dickey, L.D. (Ed.): *Clinical Ecology*, Springfield, Thomas, 1976, p. 306.
3. Carl C. Pfeiffer, pp. 11, 12, and 377.
   "On the origin of cancer cells" by Otto Warburg in *Science Journal*, February 1956, pp. 309-314.
4. Deming, *Water: The Fountain of Opportunity*, pp. 5 and 14.

5. Pfeiffer, Carl C.: *Mental & Elemental Nutrition.* New Canaan, Connecticut, Keats, 1975, pp. 331-332.
6. *Encyclopedia Britannica,* 1967, s.v. Water.
7. Kingzett's Chemical Encyclopedia, s.v. Water.
8. Deming, *Water: The Fountain of Opportunity,* p. 97.
9. Andrews, William A., et al.: *Freshwater Ecology.* Englewood, New Jersey, P-H, 1972, p. viii.
10. Andrews, et al., *Freshwater Ecology,* p. 344.
11. Andrews, et al., *Freshwater Ecology.*
12. *Environmental Science & Technology,* July 1977, p. 661.
13. *Environmental Science & Technology,* April 1977, pp. 342-347.
Environmental Science & Technology, July 1977, pp. 660-665.
14. Pfeiffer, *Mental & Elemental Nutrition,* pp. 329-332.
15. Nikel, C.M.: *Breathing for Survival.* Hicksville, New York, Exposition, 1975, p. 26.
16. Silver, Francis V.: Personal communication to the author.

Recommended Additional Reading

Biological Problems in Water Pollution, transactions of the 1959 Seminar, Technical Report W60-3 (1960). Available from the United States Department of Health, Education, and Welfare, Public Health Service.

Chapter 14

THE OASIS

GUY O. PFEIFFER

"**R**EPETITION makes the model student." The words of a professor forty years ago are still of current value. Repetition of ideas in this volume may aid you in understanding, finding, and treating your chronic illness and lead you to an oasis of relief.

In this chapter, an oasis will be constructed that the chronically ill individual may enter to rest whenever the chemicals in the atmosphere at work, at play, or even in the dwelling, begin to affect the sense of well-being.

Time and time again it has been determined that a restful period in a "less contaminated" area will bring about the ability of the individual to function normally in a full-time endeavor. With this premise in mind, it is often acceptable to construct a single area that is less contaminated rather than to attempt to construct a completely new residence. The professional individual will have the private office, the conference room, or another area converted into an oasis so that he is able to function at peak levels.

The Occupational Safety and Health Administration (OSHA) decrees that certain minimum standards be met in all commercial and manufacturing work places. This, indeed, is striving for an "oasis" of safety when compared with working conditions in earlier years. However, the required minimum standards of OSHA will not meet the rigid standards we must maintain to attempt to aid the chronically ill patient.

The examination rooms, the waiting rooms, and the treatment rooms of the allergist or the clinical ecologist should also be constructed so that an oasis effect is obtained. It is impractical to attempt to control the odors of the individual, of his clothing, or of his tobacco and perfumes in the halls of commerce. But it is not only possible, but mandatory, that those individuals who seek aid and thus enter into a physician's office complex be quickly advised that they are entering a less contaminated area and must be as free as possible of any chemical odors. By their unsuspected odors, they might influence the examination of fellow patients.

The oasis may be a temporary affair. Without major change of construction, often a trial oasis can be developed. By new construction or remodeling, a permanent oasis can be developed. Repetition of many ideas presented in Chapter 12 by Mr. Silver in his discussion of the ecology of household supplies and how to clean up an area is considered to be worthwhile at this time.

THE TRIAL OR TEMPORARY OASIS

In order to develop the oasis many factors are involved. A room with a single door to other parts of the residence is much superior to a room with connecting doors to other rooms. A clothes closet for storage may or may not be advisable. To develop a temporary oasis let us proceed step by step:

1. Empty the room that is going to be involved. All furniture, all floor coverings, drapes, pictures, etc. are completely removed. Cleaning of this room is the next step. Cleaning solution that the individual can tolerate is used. Sprays of any type, phenol-type products, and any scented products must not be used. The ceiling and the walls are then again carefully examined. If the odor of paint or insecticide additives are noted, this room may not be as good as another room in this residence. If odors of this type are found, the outgassing will probably continue for months or years. If another room is not available, some method of removing odors of paints should be followed. Increasing outgassing of any product is by the use of elevated heat. A room that has been painted long ago seldom presents the problem that is found in a newly painted area. To quickly "age" the area, we have found heating the sealed area to 80°F for seven to ten days followed by ventilating the area for eight hours to be effective. This procedure produces a usable area. To alleviate the outgassing from paints, one might use low volatility painting materials, which will shorten the outgassing

period, and it may tend toward lesser outgassing at the lower comfort temperature levels. Filtration of air may be used in dealing with this problem and will be discussed later. While thinking of odors from the walls, it must be stressed that sleeping or resting should never be done with the head against the wall or in the corner of the room.

2. Ceiling light fixtures, as well as floor lamps and table lamps, must be examined. Plastic shades, when warm, may give off toxic chemical gases. For this reason, glass or cotton shades are superior. If it is possible, fluorescent lighting is considered to be superior to incandescent lighting. The incandescent bulb becomes hot. If dust is floating in the air and it touches the hot light bulb, it will be charred and, thus, be converted into fried dust. The temperature of a fluorescent bulb is never more than warm.

3. Before pictures, mirrors, wall plaques are returned to the room, they must be closely inspected. Glues that may or may not have an odor are often suspect. Again, aging for increased outgassing may be sufficient. Screws or nails are much better for use. All plastic coverings, frames, and any other knick-knacks are suspect items. Rays of sunlight reaching these objects, the oils used in the paintings, and the varnish used on the picture frames are able to outgas and may produce illness in the sensitive individual. It is better to keep the object out of the room than to take a chance by bringing it in and finally find that it can produce problems.

4. It is suggested that, instead of having drab or unsightly walls, mirrors, ceramics, tile, and china objects be artfully installed by suspension on hooks. Use of any adhesives is not recommended, however, lest outgassing of such items would incite undesirable symptoms of illness.

5. The windows are important for many reasons. A view of the outside is often good *psychotherapy* for the room-bound individual. A colored plastic sheeting applied to the outside of the window glass will reduce the glare. It will also reduce the heat to the curtains and drapes, if they are exposed to direct sunlight. These curtains and drapes should be decorated with vegetable dye colors. Chemical dyes may be a problem. The material should be of organic fiber, such as nonsynthetic burlap, cotton, or silk. Cellular rayon also seems to be of

little problem. Synthetic products, as a group, are highly suspect.

6. All floor coverings are suspect. Before returning any floor coverings to this room, it is well to refinish the floor, let it air out, gas out, and then use cotton throw rugs. These cotton throw rugs can be tumbled or washed frequently. Vegetable dye wool rugs are acceptable to most individuals. The only rugs that fit this specification are the natural dye, handcarded, spun, and hand-woven Navajo and *Hopi rugs*. These, by current economic standards, are very expensive. Old Oriental rugs are also occasionally acceptable. More recently produced Oriental rugs are being colored with synthetic dye, which makes such rugs useless for hypersensitive individuals.

7. The woodwork of the doors, jambs, window trim, and floor presents a problem. To finish or refinish this woodwork, there are two advised methods. The first, which is more sturdy, is also more problem to produce; this is the use of varnish. The alternate heating and airing of the area for many weeks will hasten the outgassing until it is acceptable to most individuals. The second method of refinishing is by the use of shellac. Shellac is mixed with synthetic ethyl alcohol. This is very toxic to chemically sensitive individuals; however, usually within ten days after application, the outgassing is complete and is acceptable to most individuals.

8. Brick, tile, or ceramic floors are usually acceptable. Unpainted concrete floors, for some unexplained reason, produce problems. Linoleum coverings with their hard base are acceptable to most individuals. Vinyl floors are better in sheet form than in small tiled sections. The glues used on these are always suspect. The synthetic indoor-outdoor type of carpet is also highly suspect.

When changing a temporary oasis to a permanent oasis, many of these ideas can be incorporated so that the completed product is attractive, as well as practical, to the chronically ill individual.

THERMAL CONTROL

Heating

Before reintroducing any article into the room, a most important procedure must be carried out. It may require modification of the heating system. The room will probably have one or more air ducts. Some of these air ducts will bring the air into the room. Others will carry the air from the room and direct the air to the furnace where it is again heated. The sealing off of these ducts is most important as this oasis must be isolated as much as possible from airborne products from other parts of the residence or the building. The following suggestions may be of help.

The closure of these intake and return air ducts is usually quite simple. The duct plate or louvre is removed. Nonglazed, nonwaxed, white, sturdy package paper is cut to size and placed over the duct entry or exit. The louvre is then replaced. Usually no air motion can be found when the furnace fan is on in this area. Printed newspapers are not recommended because of the printing dyes. Unprinted paper can be used. The paper should not be taped over the louvre because of possible glue exposure. Also, the glue may disfigure the wall or floor when it is removed. The outlet port is covered, as well as the inlet port. The inlet port must be covered because the return air duct might pull air from under the door into the clean room and, thus, into the return air duct. With this duct properly sealed, there will be less negative pressure in the oasis room.

Solar heating of this oasis is the method of choice; however, even in southern states, it has been found that auxiliary heat is needed 25 percent or more of the heating period due to the limitation of our present technology and economics. The next-best method of satisfactory heating is the portable *hot water electric heater*. No electrical resistance heating units are recommended.

Cooling

The method of cooling recommended is the window-type air conditioner. Only filtered air is brought into the oasis area. Many individuals, however, have determined that they can tolerate central air conditioning. If the individual can tolerate central air conditioning, the covers that had been placed over the intake and output vents may now be removed; the ducts, which have been inactive, must now be cleansed by careful vacuuming. If central air conditioning is being used, the door of the room can then be kept open as much as the individual wishes.

Filtration

Proper filters in the air conditioner may be adequate for comfort in the oasis. At times, a portable ambient chemical extraction (*A.C.E.*) filtration system must be added to this area. Depending upon the sensitivities of the individual, charcoal, or Purafil filters, or combinations of these may be of value. The specific type of filter is very important and is discussed in Chapter 11.

FURNISHINGS

The contents of the oasis must be under constant surveillance. Offending items can be removed before causing extensive problems. Remember, each and every item brought into the oasis is suspect.

Bed Frames

The ultimate goal is comfort. However, it must be acceptable to the individual with chronic illness. The bed frame must be inspected for any odor from fresh paints, plasticizers, oils, and cleansing materials. Synthetic, or even some tanned leather, headboards outgas and produce many bizarre problems. Metal or wood frames are usually best. Freshly glued parts may be a source of problem.

Springs, Mattress, and Pillows

Covered springs are usually acceptable but must be carefully examined. The coverings of the springs on which the mattress rests is usually far enough away from the individual so that problems are at a minimum. If severe problems occur, the patient should have this unit custom-made with acceptable products. The mattress and the pillow deserve much attention. Neither must be offensive to the patient. Many so-called cotton mattresses have a foam blanket covering the innersprings or attached to the mattress covering. Since 1972 the flammability standards for mattresses have dictated that mattresses meet certain requirements. These requirements make mattresses unacceptable to many chemically hypersensitive individuals. A layer of foam or synthetic material placed under the mattress cover on the sleeping surface is usually the offending agent. In a short time, outgassing is noted and illness increases in the sensitive individual. The foam rubber or synthetic mattress, as a substitute, is not advised.

Lying on a troublesome pillow may produce many restless hours. A plastic pillow cover is not recommended. The pillow case must be one that produces no symptoms in the patient. The pillow itself should not be made of synthetic materials. If a synthetic pillow is used, the individual should ever be alert to the fact that if problems arise, he should change pillows for a trial period. Many individuals find a rolled-up cotton blanket acceptable when it is inserted into the pillow case. Most individuals can tolerate a feather or down pillow. It is believed that the feathers are not the allergic problem as much as it is the mold and mold spores that develop in the feathers. With this in mind, the care of the cotton or feather pillow is quite simple. The pillow is inserted into the clothes dryer and tumbled at low heat at weekly or even more frequent intervals.

Bed Linens

Linens are somewhat difficult to obtain. Permanent-pressed cottons should be washed repeatedly before using. Cellular rayons are often well tolerated. Part-cotton acrylics, acetates, etc. are often totally unacceptable. Blankets are also of many types. Handmade quilts are sometimes a source of problems. Synthetic fillers instead of cotton fillers may be troublesome. Synthetic patches may also be viewed with suspicion. Cotton and wool blankets often are acceptable. Synthetics, again, are viewed with suspicion. Bedspreads should be of cotton or cellular rayon. Brilliant synthetic dyes are extremely suspect.

Other furnishings of the oasis are chosen one by one. Chairs must be suspected of glue odors. Synthetic or leather tanning chemicals must be tested for outgassing. The dressing table and its contents are also highly suspect. Cosmetics of any type should not be used in the oasis. Chests of drawers are also chosen with care because of the glue, varnish, and resin wood used for their construction. Clothing must also be of such material as to be noncontributory to chronic illness.

Knickknacks

Play toys, stuffed animals, school pennants, and other items of this class of materials are chosen, inspected, and added one at a time after the use of this bare room has proven that the individual is improved when using his oasis.

Scented soaps, cosmetics, cleansing products, dry cleaning materials, candles, incense, detergents, and each and every article must all be evaluated. Even a slightly suspicious item should not be used on the clothing, walls, or floors.

There is an individual variation encountered in the use of radio or TV in the oasis. Again, an individual evaluation is made by the chronically ill patient. The warm air emanating from such appliances may incite symptoms of illness. (*See* Dr. Byrd's report on this in Chapter 16 of this book.)

Cleaning of the oasis and the bathroom that is used by the individual should be governed by the principles outlined in Chapter 12.

Visitors to the room are often a problem. It is most important that the individual who must seek relief in the oasis, while being tactful, must be very firm and allow no visitors to enter his oasis if he is able to sense any odors emanating from the visitor. Such odors consist of smoke, cosmetics, or clothing odors acquired through cleaning or saturation at work.

The Clothing and Storage Closet

The long-term storage of articles is often a problem. It is easy to forget what is stored in them. It is best to recheck and evict as much as is needed. Clothing that is a potential problem is not kept in this room, even though it is worn by the individual in his workaday world. Oils, such as gun oil, the oil-treated fishing gear, firearms and other sporting equipment, and cleaning material are all suspect and must be individually evaluated by the patient before inclusion in the oasis. Do not accumulate reading material in the patient's room. Ink outgasses. It has been suggested that an ultraviolet light be placed in the closet, which might inhibit molds and their associated problems. The ultraviolet lamp is not without danger. The production of ozone tends to be increased in ultraviolet lighting. The use of inert mold inhibitors is also of value. Impregon Liquid® has aided in this regard.

EXECUTIVE OASIS

The executive oasis is treated in much the same manner as the temporary domiciliary oasis, except that a careful survey must be made of all products in the executive suite. There should be filters, as discussed in the chapter on air filtration, operating on a twenty-four-hour basis in this suite. The mimeographed material, mail, various papers, inks, etc. must be carefully evaluated. It has been said that the executive oasis must be kept more orderly than the usual executive office in that the outgassing of papers, letters, newspapers, magazines, etc. is a much more serious problem than is commonly believed.

As much as possible, storage of material, as in the filing cabinet, should be kept in another room and not in the oasis.

Some method to alert visitors, other than the absence of ashtrays, must be developed so that this oasis is not contaminated by tobacco smoke. Major conferences, if possible, should be held in another room and not in the executive oasis; however, if this is impractical, then there should be an increase in the filtration of the air by specially engineered filters. The thermal control of this room should be carried out in a similar manner as in the domestic oasis.

The cleaning of this room by the janitor demands a special

procedure for the janitor to follow. The cleaning materials and cleaning equipment used should be kept separate from those materials used for the other parts of the building. This is necessary, as these cleaning materials and cleaning equipment can become contaminated with inciteful chemicals used elsewhere. The oasis, as well as the areas immediately adjacent to the oasis, should not use chemical deodorants or air fresheners.

The opening and closing of windows to allow outdoor air into this area may or may not be allowed, depending upon the location of the oasis and the pollution factor in the outside air.

THE PERMANENT OASIS

This room is designed by applying construction hints as listed in this volume. Before constructing a permanent oasis, the establishing of relief from symptoms of the individual in a temporary oasis is important. Why should you build a permanent change into your building if you have not materially improved in such an oasis?

The Ideal Dwelling

This discussion is presented in order that the hypersensitive individual can logically develop an area in which he can live more comfortably in this highly polluted civilization. The single dwelling, whether it be a mobile home or a standard structure, can be developed or remodeled to produce improved living conditions. The multiple family-type dwelling, whether it be apartment, townhouse, condominium, flat, or penthouse, can present special problems. Your neighbors above, below, or to one side of you can, through their use of insecticides, sprays, paints, and all cleaning equipment, cause a continual problem to you by the seepage of these contaminants into your "clean air." It is similar to the oasis that is not as efficient as the entire dwelling being constructed according to the principles of clinical ecology. Admittedly, an oasis may not be the ideal dwelling; however, it does provide early relief, and it also provides the experience upon which a permanent dwelling can be developed at minimal cost of untried changes.

In conclusion, it is well to repeat that the garage should not be attached to the building where the oasis is located. The outgassing of stored paint cans, oils, gasoline, and oil drippings on the floor will often produce problems in the less contaminated area. Many times there is special construction between the garage or the storage area of such materials; however, transfer of the outgassing by way of the attic may be found and the patient may continue to have problems.

The testing of suspected items is carried out by many methods:

1. The sniffing or smelling of the suspected product will often tell the individual whether he will probably be able to accept the product in the oasis.

2. The sense of touch may also impart to the individual his acceptance or denial of the product. It is well known that the wine taster and wine sniffer can tell the excellence or the quality of the wine. It is the same with the sense of feel. Many individuals, by sitting on a product or by feeling the product, will soon experience strange sensations. This has proven to be a very accurate method of separating a product that is tolerated from a product that is not tolerated by the individual.

3. A small portion of the product can be placed in a glass jar, sealed, and baked at 350° for two hours. Upon cooling, the seal is broken and the individual can sniff the jar immediately upon opening it. If it is intolerable, then it should never be used in the oasis area.

Chapter 15

REMODELING AN EXISTING HOUSE FOR THE HYPERSENSITIVE

JOHN W. ARGABRITE

FOR the purpose of this chapter, a hypersensitive individual is one who is sensitive to either or both of the gaseous and particulate content of domiciliary air. This chapter, therefore, will consider numerous factors that must be taken into consideration when remodeling an existing structure. Such remodeling is intended to aid the hypersensitive individual with his health problems associated with environmental influences. An important factor, and a difficult situation to correct, is comfort control. This is due to the fact that many structures use a hot air ducted furnace system. The furnace in such a system may create two principal types of *pollution* in the domiciliary air:

1. As fossil fuel has usually been used in this furnace, there is a tendency to leak both raw fuel and products of combustion into the ambient air, despite carefully engineered precautions to prevent such a possibility.
2. The furnace heats the domiciliary air by passing it over a high-temperature heat exchanger. As the dust particles in the air cross the heat exchanger, they are carbonized and thus release minute amounts of gaseous chemicals into the domiciliary air.

With modern technology many of these products can be measured; however, some by-products cannot be precisely evaluated. Clinically it has been established that these various contaminants can bring about chemically induced chronic illness to the hypersensitive individual.

When the remodeling project is being considered, it can thus be understood that the heating system must be redesigned to prevent the two potential threats of air pollution within the house. The redesigned system proposed in this paper is rather expensive. Therefore, it is suggested that the hypersensitive individual first test himself by the "oasis" principle as is explained in Chapter 14 of this volume. If such a test proves to be helpful to the health of the hypersensitive individual, the remodeling of the hot air duct system is then recommended.

REMODELING A HOT AIR
DUCTED FURNACE SYSTEM

If the homeowner decides to retain the duct portion of the system in his remodeling, an early step will be the replacement of the furnace with a thermal chamber, which is illustrated in Figure 15-1. It will be noted here that the air is heated and cooled through individual coils. These coils are filled with liquids thermally conditioned only to a moderate degree. This liquid is heated or cooled in a burner unit building (BUB), which is completely removed from the house. This prevents gaseous contamination of the domiciliary air. The air can be conditioned by one of several different ways:

1. The liquid at the BUB can be heated by a conventional boiler, and it is then transferred through pipes with a circulating pump to and through the heating coil in the thermal chamber, which is located in the basement of the house. This boiler system requires maintaining temperatures of the liquid under 220°F. This temperature level is critical in order to prevent carbonizing of microscopic dust particles in the domiciliary air as it passes over the coils in the thermal chamber.

If a boiler is used for heating, then the cooling coil in the thermal chamber can be supplied with chilling liquid from one of two sources:

A. A deep well generally provides water cool enough to chill the domiciliary air needed for comfort levels. This water also is circulated with a pump through the cooling coil in the thermal chamber, similar to the heating-liquid circulating method.

B. If no deep-well water is available, then a conventional Freon-gas air conditioner can be used to chill the water

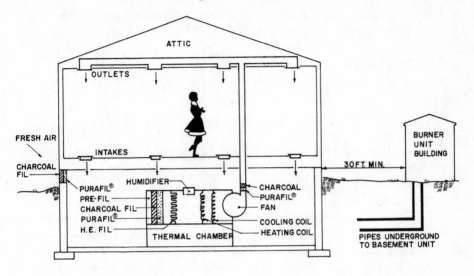

Figure 15-1.

for supplying the cooling coil in the thermal chamber. It is important, however, to locate the air conditioner at the BUB in order to prevent any contamination of the domiciliary air with Freon gas.

2. Another method for heating and cooling is the use of the Amana® heat transfer module (HTM). The convenience of this HTM unit is in its capability of handling the liquid for both coils in the thermal chamber. By reversing the heating process of the HTM unit, the liquid in the system can be cooled. This eliminates the necessity of two systems, as in the case of the boiler and the deep-well water supply. The mechanical principles of the HTM system are interesting, but they will not be discussed here. However, the HTM must be located at the BUB regardless of the type of fuel that is used, because of the potential for Freon gas leakage and it polluting the domiciliary air.

3. One more method that can supply heating and cooling liquid for the thermal chamber is a specially designed heat pump. This type of heat pump is described in Chapter 9. The author of that chapter and I remodeled a structure based on the principles illustrated by Figure 15-1. This

system uses a very low heating-liquid temperature and requires a constant running air-circulating fan. The sound from this fan evokes some criticism. However, most of the hum can be filtered or dampened by proper insulation.

CLEANING THE AIR IN A DUCT SYSTEM

A study of Figure 15-1, of the proposed heating and cooling system, illustrates that the thermal chamber includes several stages of air filtration. This filtration is needed, as other pollutions than those created by the furnace can bring about health problems to a hypersensitive individual. It will also be noted that in order to assure an adequate supply of domiciliary air, an outdoor-air intake is provided. This will assure an adequate amount of oxygenated air. A filter at the outdoor-air intake consists of an activated charcoal cell and a Purafil cell. These two cells have the ability of removing several hundred different gaseous chemicals, thereby assuring the maximum protection from both automotive and other pollutants, which are present in the ambient air of the cleanest modern communities.

The provision of air depollution at the outdoor-air intake at the basement location is not usually adequate for the continued health of the hypersensitive individual. Profuse pollution occurs from the living activities in the upper area of the home. Some of these sources are human metabolism; cooking fumes; cleaning fumes; bathroom odors, as well as backdrafted fumes from drains; cosmetic odors; and outgassing from synthetic fabrics and upholstery. This pollution from the living activities is so much greater than the outdoor pollution that a very sophisticated depollution arrangement is needed in this unit. A prefilter is needed, before the charcoal and Purafil cells, due to the gross lint and foot-traffic dusts that are present in all homes. To assure that no fine dust passes through the charcoal and Purafil cells into the heated air, a high efficiency (HE) filter is provided on the downstream side. This is usually 4 to 6 inches thick, and the filter media is shaped in a series of "V" forms in order to maximize the filtration area of the air passing through it.

Following such meticulous depollution, it would seem that no additional depollution would be needed. This is not entirely true. The fan system is also a source of pollution. To combat this, another activated charcoal and Purafil cell installation is provided in the air supply riser.

With the isolation of the thermal conditioning units at the BUB and the thorough air depollution at the thermal chamber in the basement of the house, the ambient air should be tolerable to the hypersensitive individual.

REMODELING THE NONDUCTED HOUSE

There are several electrical heating systems that can be employed to provide heat in an existing house which does not have ducts for air distribution. Each of these systems has some disadvantages for the hypersensitive individual. The most desirable of the electric heating system is Intertherm. It utilizes a baseboard module. The module incorporates hermetically sealed water with antifreeze, which is heated by an electric element inside a copper pipe. The surface of this pipe does not exceed 220°F, which prevents carbonizing of house dust in the air that passes across the heating parts of the Intertherm module.

Intertherm also has an air conditioning unit to complement the heating system with an air-cooling service. Although the compressor and chilling unit of this system consists of moving parts and Freon gas, it is designed for easy installation on the outside of the house. The conventional ducts are replaced with a dropped-ceiling plenum. A simple installation, employing this concept, is illustrated in Figure 15-2.

The Intertherm heating system and air-cooling system can be supplemented with a portable air depollution unit. The Air Conditioning Engineers Company of Decatur, Illinois manufactures such a depollution unit. It is housed in a steel cabinet, with baked-on finish. Most hypersensitive individuals experience good results with the A.C.E. depollution. The units can be custom-designed to the most demanding requirements for air cleanliness. Therefore, with the clean heat input by the

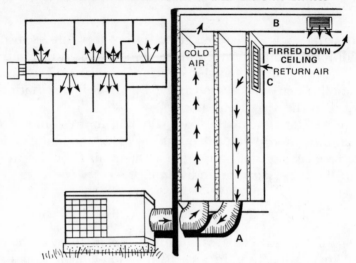

Filtered air is drawn through 12" flexible, insulated round ducts (A) into the unit where it is dehumidified and cooled to provide soft, gentle air conditioning throughout the home.

There is absolutely no energy loss created by heat from a blower motor within the building such as that which normally occurs with other air conditioners (and adds to air conditioning load up to 40,000 Btuh per day). Neither is any energy lost through ducts in the basements or in high temperature attics which can increase cooling costs up to 20% or more. . . especially important with today's increased electricity costs.

The illustration above shows a false ceiling (B) in the hallway 8" to 10" below the regular ceiling. Outlet grilles (C) are placed above the doors of each room. To circulate cool air to rooms not connected to a hallway, it is recommended that a firred down, false ceiling be used.

It is then a simple matter to extend the firred down false ceiling distributing system, as shown, to a cool air riser (normally the width of a closet by 12" to accommodate the round duct from the air conditioner). The ducts are wedged in at the base or sides of the cool air riser, whichever is most convenient. (Please note: It is most important that construction tape be used where panels or duct tube join together to avoid losss of energy).

An additional riser approximately 12" x the width of the closet must then be provided to run from the floor where the tube from the return opening of the air conditioner is connected to an air filtering grille located as near the ceiling as possible.

The Intertherm SCH air conditioner is placed on a concrete slab approximately 12" from the building so that both cool and warm air insulated ducts can readily be connected to risers in the building.

For buildings of two or more stories, this same procedure should be followed, using separate units wherever possible for zoning control of bedroom vs. living area for maximum comfort and lowest cooling costs.

Figure 15-2.

Intertherm system, and by depollution with an A.C.E., system, the hypersensitive individual will find his remodeled house reasonably tolerable.

SUNDRY FEATURES, FURNISHINGS, AND FOMENTATION

Humidity

To control humidity with a central duct system using a heat exchanger, have the humidifier placed in the thermal chamber just before or just after the heating coils. To reduce probable mold growth, use a 5 micron nylon filter, which will remove most of the molds from passing into the environment. Floor model humidifying units are acceptable, but they must be cleaned periodically to control the thermophilic molds. Another method for humidification is the use of a metal pan below a white Turkish towel that is suspended from the ceiling. This acts as a wick. It is a good humidifier that results in a minimum of problems with mold growth (1). (Fig. 15-3)

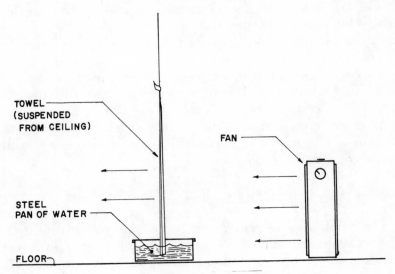

TOWEL
(SUSPENDED
FROM CEILING)

FAN

STEEL
PAN OF WATER

FLOOR

Figure 15-3.

Ventilation

It is important to provide a good outside source of air. Without a doubt there is no substitute for unpolluted ambient air. It is preferred that the air intake be installed away from the garage, chimney, and other polluting conditions such as heavy traffic and activities involving the use of fertilizers, fungicides, and pesticides. If outside pollution is unavoidable, then any air taken in from the outside should be treated with a charcoal and Purafil depollution unit.

The use of an exhaust fan is also important for proper ventilation. It is generally accepted that even the best insulated home undergoes air infiltration that produces approximately one change of total air each hour. However, if heavy indoor-originated pollution needs to be removed quickly, a good exhaust fan becomes indispensable. Such a fan should not be operated indefinitely because it can create a negative indoor pressure resulting in backdrafting of fireplaces or increased load on the fan motor.

Kitchen

The best floor covering is ceramic tile. It is not too practical with children on the premises, however, as anything that is dropped usually breaks. It emits no odors and is easy to clean. Linoleum is also good and is self-polishing. Vinyl tile and sheet vinyl floor covering are good. The glue used for the vinyl tiles and floor covering is extremely offensive, but it only outgasses for about twenty-four hours. There is also a hard plastic hypoxy floor, which is suitable; it outgasses for about two weeks. One could use hardwood floors (prefinished) with cotton or wool throw rugs.

Appliances

Gas appliances should never be considered for use in the chemically sensitive person's home. A suitable range hood with an exhaust fan for an electric cooking stove is excellent. The range hood is necessary to remove cooking odors and odors from self-cleaning ovens. Corning® ceramic stoves are easy to clean. Extremely sensitive patients may use electronic radar ovens. At the present time, I feel that the absence of charring the food, the preservation of vitamins and nutrients in the food, plus the speed in serving time, far outweigh the potential hazard of radiation. Electronic ovens give off odors of cooking, so an exhaust fan in this area is mandatory. People with cardiac pacemakers manufactured five or six years ago may have problems with electronic ovens. This is not true of the newer cardiac pacemakers.

In a home without central air conditioning, there should be a sufficient size wall- or window-type air conditioner for the kitchen. This extra size is needed in order to take care of the extra heat generated by cooking. For fast venting of odors from cooking and those odors produced by the self-cleaning oven, a fan should be installed in close proximity to this area.

Kitchen cupboards should be prefinished. Food supplies such as flour, sugar, and corn meal should be stored in metal or glass containers. This discourages insects and rodents. It also prevents possible absorption of fumes from the plastic containers.

Gas refrigerators and other gas appliances are strongly condemned in the home of the chemically sensitive person. It is now rather difficult to obtain a refrigerator that is not self-defrosting. The heat cycle combined with the plastic liner of the refrigerator gives off fumes. We have found that this often contaminates the food and the ice cubes. The containers in the icebox should be of glass or stainless steel to minimize this problem. The soft plastic food storage vessels are not advocated.

Illumination of the kitchen is important. It is suggested that Vita-lite® fluorescent lights be used (2). Vita lites are slightly more expensive but have a much longer service life. The manufacturer states that they are a full-spectrum light, which includes ultraviolet light that is thought by many to be beneficial to health. Conventional lights emit infrared but little or no ultraviolet light (3).

Again, I repeat, the cooking and dining area should be well

ventilated to minimize the troublesome effect of cooking fumes traveling to the other parts of the home and especially into the sleeping area.

Garage

The garage should be spaced away from the house. If a connection to the house is wanted, a breezeway is acceptable. This tends to keep the fumes from the gasoline vehicle and other items stored in the garage from entering into the house. In the event that your home has a flat roof with a connected garage, there are some methods by which fumes entering the house can be decreased. A series of double doors with a hallway to trap the outside air from entering the home may be possible. If the home has a connected garage, a hip roof, and an attic, a shield must be placed at the junction point and the garage attic be completely sealed from the house attic. A possible method to use for this situation is a shield of wood with fiberglass insulation on each side of the wood wall and aluminum paper over the insulation. It is important that negative pressure never be made in the attic in a house with this situation, as it will then pull air from the garage side of the attic.

Storage spaces in the garage should be cupboards or wood chests that can be closed. These are good places to store old cans of paint and other chemical items. This does not prevent outgassing but seems to contain the odors in a small area, and, thus, the odors are not noticed as much in the adjacent living areas.

The garage should never be under the house, as there is no way to seal off and control the fumes from filtering through the floor into the living area.

Attic

Be sure the duct system is metal and the joints and connections are sound, for in the event of any leak, this will act as a vacuum bringing offensive air into the home. All attics should have a thermostatically controlled exhaust fan to remove hot air, which also reduces the fire hazard.

Utilities

Hot water heater, washer, and dryer, which are all electric, should be set aside from the main part of the home or put in the basement under the kitchen to confine odors to one section of the home. Be sure to have the dryer vented to the outside. In addition, install an exhaust system to remove detergent odor. Gas-fired hot water heaters are not recommended because the pilot light frequently outgasses. Gas-fired dryers are not recommended for the same reasons. They also contaminate the clothes with gas fumes.

Bathroom

It is best to have one outside wall with a window plus an exhaust fan to remove odors. Sears manufactures a toilet under the trade name Airo Magic®, which acts as a vacuum to remove odors when it is flushed.

Many of the new light fixtures are fitted with a fan, which operates off the light switch; this activates the fan when the light is turned on.

Clothing Closets

Closets should be equipped with an exhaust system to remove dry cleaning fumes. An effective ventilation system requires a fan that exhausts to the outside. The replacement air can be drawn into the closet under the door from the adjacent room. If the room air has been treated with a depollution unit, the clothing in the closet will be freshened substantially.

Be sure that the closed door fits snugly. If the closet does not have a door, be sure that one is installed. Such a door closure should provide about a one-half-inch space between the floor and the bottom of the door, so air can pass thru the closet when the exhaust fan is running.

Living Room with a Fireplace

Be sure to have a glass screen in front of the fireplace — one which provides a damper at the bottom of the screen. Such a screen minimizes the heat loss up the chimney when the fireplace is inoperative. It also protects against down drafts through the fireplace. A fireplace has many disadvantages, such as excessive heat loss, high pollution input, consumption of oxygen from the inside ambient space, decreasing inside humidity, and backdrafting fumes into the room. Outside air can be brought directly to the front of the fireplace but behind the glass doors. This will decrease the possibility of backdrafting. A hypersensitive individual would be advised to avoid the disadvantages of a fireplace.

Floor and Wall Treatment

Carpeting for the chemically sensitive person should be wool with Wilton weave preferred. Such a carpet should not have a rubberized back. Do not use rubber padding, as it never ceases to outgas. Jute padding is recommended for use under carpeting for the chemically sensitive person. For those who are sensitive to woolen particles, an air depollution machine is recommended. If possible, a central vacuum cleaning system should be installed to minimize dust pollution. Tank-type and upright vacuum cleaners should not be used, because they create dust pollution and their motors give off oil fumes that are offensive to the chemically sensitive person.

Wood paneling for the walls is acceptable, but be sure not to use cedar or pine. Cedar gives off its fumes in the form of an odor, and the knots in pine give off a resin, both of which can be offensive to the hypersensitive person. A low-pollution sealer applied to pine wood may make it tolerable to some individuals. Fir is a wood that gives off minimally offensive fumes. Most hardwood paneling is tolerable to hypersensitives, but it is substantially more costly than the soft woods.

Illumination

The living room should be well lighted with large Thermopane windows in order to provide ample daylight and to act as a source of solar heat during the winter period. Locating the windows to the south and east will conserve heat, and protect against the prevailing northwest winds. A good window casing is metal, but it is expensive and not too practical since it causes heavy heat loss.

Bedrooms

Wooden floors with throw rugs of cotton or wool are usually least bothersome to the chemically sensitive. If the bathroom is connected to the bedroom, an adequate exhaust fan is essential; however, all bathrooms should have exhaust systems.

Basement Recreational Room

The use of vinyl, which is a self-polishing tile, sheet vinyl floor covering, or linoleum is simple to clean and does not outgas extensively. Hardwood floors are acceptable in the basement but require a great deal more upkeep. There is also the potential that the humidity will be higher in the basement, and the increased growth of molds are more difficult to control with a wood floor. A dehumidifier is often indicated for use in the basement.

Painting

The chemically sensitive individual usually finds that indoor paints might be either acrylic or cassinate paint. The individual should have a test strip of the paint to find whether or not he can tolerate such a specific paint. The most expensive, and probably the best, interior wall covering is troweled plaster. Craftsmen who apply the plaster are becoming increasingly difficult to obtain. One should avoid plaster that contains certain synthetic plastics or chemical treatment for fireproofing and mold retardation.

Floors

The refinishing of floors also is very important to consider. Shellac apparently produces less trouble than varnish. Varnish produces less trouble than the synthetic enamels. The shellac that is suspended in hydrocarbon ethanol or synthetic alcohol will outgas in approximately one week. Varnish may take two to three weeks, and the synthetic liquid often will take six weeks. For floors other than the self-polishing floor tile, a hard wax is superior to a liquid wax. The odor produced usually disappears in forty-eight hours.

Fixtures

Electrical fixtures should be limited to metal or glass. Do not use plastic, fiberglass, or plastic foam fixtures. Lacquered metal parts should be closely observed, as they tend to give off odors when warmed up. After following proper curing, they are usually tolerated by the individual.

Candles

Petroleum wax or scented candles are to be avoided. Candles that are kept available for use in possible power outages should be made of beeswax. Corningware® has a new glass floating candle that burns on vegetable oil. It has been found to be acceptable to most chemically sensitive persons.

Drapes

Drapes should be cotton, linen, or silk. The synthetics and fiberglass should be avoided. Most drapes have been previously treated with dieldrin as a pesticide, mold eradicator, and fire retardant. All of these are offensive to the chemically sensitive person. They should be avoided. Drapes should be custom-made from nontreated materials.

Wallpaper

Wallpaper can be offensive to the chemically sensitive individual. The wallpaper paste may be a mold-growing media. There are many different types of wallpaper, some with acrylic paint and rice paper, which can be offensive to the sensitive person. One can make his own paste using flour, water and calcium propinate as a mold preventor. One should test the wallpaper before it is applied.

Wallboard

Wallboard has a fire proofing chemical added to its structure that is offensive to many chemically sensitive individuals. Painting the wallboard with acrylic paint does seem to help; however, this is not definite for all hypersensitives.

Roofing

Tar paper should not be used for roofs in direct contact with the board decking. This often creates a situation where there is a seeping downward of fumes when the sun heats the roof and thereby pollutes the living areas. Mylar® sheets to be used as an underlayment are preferred. However, when warm enough, the Mylar sheets can also give off fumes. Wood shakes are recommended as the outer cover for the roof instead of asphalt shingles. Clay tile and asbestos sheets of roofing are also acceptable.

Electrical Wiring

Building codes control the wiring of the house, which limits the modification of construction. Some individuals are able to tolerate Romex®, which is a plastic-covered cable. Conduit, although more expensive, gives the greatest assurance that pollution from this source will be minimal. It is advisable to restrain the use of plastic fixtures and appliances in conjunction with any electrical installation.

Miscellaneous

Macrame for decorative purposes is discouraged, since it is made of chemically treated twine. Plastic trees and various ornaments made of synthetic fabrics, and synthetic fibers, are to be avoided.

A convenient method of testing for sensitivity to various

synthetic materials is to take a piece of the suspected material and place it in a tightly closed Mason® jar then bake it at 300°F in an oven for twenty minutes. Remove it from the oven, allow it to cool, and then smell the air in the jar. If the fumes are not offensive, it suggests that you may have a high tolerance for such materials.

CONCLUSION

Although many of the foregoing suggestions and recommendations may be tedious, it is best to take adequate time in planning any change. Proper selection of materials before installation may save many dollars and countless hours of chronic illness due to unwarranted changes. In keeping with a well-known adage, an ounce of prevention is worth a pound of cure, especially if the cure is an improper type.

BIBLIOGRAPHY

1. Lockey, Steven D.: Personal communication. Lancaster, Pennsylvania.
2. Vita Lights from Durotest Co., North Bergen, N.J.
3. Ott, John N.: *Health & Light.* New York, PB, p. 185, 1976 printing.

Chapter 16

ONE PHYSICIAN'S EXPERIENCE WITH CONDITIONED AIR

Lee Roy Byrd

TWENTY years of personal observations, with little help from those working in the field of allergy or in medicine in general, led me to the realization that my multiplicity of physical ailments resulted from reactions to a wide range of chemicals, as well as from molds and foods. The chemicals noted were those arising from or occurring in both natural and man-made materials. In large part they accounted for the odor or flavor, good or bad, of these materials.

Then in 1961 came the monograph, *Human Ecology and Susceptibility to the Chemical Environment*, by Theron G. Randolph, M.D., reporting his monumental work in understanding of many human ailments as related to hypersensitivity reactions to chemicals. For the first time I had found confirmation in medical literature of many of the observations regarding myself. This led to a period of study in his hands and to awareness of my hypersensitivity to the insecticides and other chemical residues in foods, as well as the chemicals I could neither see, feel, or smell that were emanating from synthetic materials in my environment.

These chemicals causing illness were added to the already long list that included, among other things, perfumes used to scent cosmetics and many household-cleaning items; the odor of flowers, foliage of trees, and other vegetation; tobacco smoke; and air-polluting materials or chemicals arising from motor exhausts and industrial processes.

Consideration of this wide-ranging list led to my conclusion that for me there was no place to go to get away from the materials that made me sick and still make a living. Therefore, I would have to create in my living quarters an "oasis," where I might be more able to avoid the materials that produced illness.

Also, I would need to regulate the environment in which I worked as well as I could. By these means, although all illness would not be eliminated, the degree of illness could be kept within the bounds of toleration most of the time. To accomplish this, I have found helpful a combination of systems: (1) central conditioning of air for heating and cooling, (2) window-type air cooling units or single room applications, (3) portable hot water electric heaters for single room applications, (4) an activated charcoal air filtration in central air handler, in personal respirators, and in single room respirators.

I set out to apply the oasis concept to a major portion of my home. Because of the odors and chemicals related to them, the kitchen and utility areas, the den, and guest bedroom were separated from my living area by tight-fitting, weather-stripped doors, and these spaces were air conditioned by completely separate conventional units.

In my living-dining-bedroom area, first consideration was given to providing a space with finishes and furnishings suitable for the person with hypersensitivity to chemicals. This required the use of specially selected materials, as set out in other sections of this book. Smoking and perfume-scented materials were not allowed in the area. Only my tolerated foods were served in the dining area. In addition, all openings in the building were made as close fitting as possible to reduce air leakage from outside into the living space to a bare minimum. Central air treatment was then installed in this living space to maintain temperatures at a comfortable level.

CENTRAL AIR TREATMENT

As plans were worked out for installation of a central air treatment system many problems became apparent. In such systems as usually installed, it was found that many factors are harmful to an individual hypersensitive to chemicals, such as the following:

1. The plenum and air-return portions of the duct system were lined inside with fiberglass mats glued in place for air-noise control and heat insulation. This fiberglass consisted of glass fibers bonded together with a plastic to

form a mat. This contributed as pollutants to the air stream the chemicals emanated by the plastic and glue.

2. Heating was carried out in many units with resistance electric coils or natural gas burners.

3. Under the cooling coils for catching the condensate was a metal drip pan coated with wax of petroleum origin as a rust preventative.

4. The side and top panels of the air handler (cooling-heating coils and blower) unit were lined with fiberglass mats glued in place.

5. The electric motor for the squirrel cage fan blower was located inside the unit, thus exposing the air stream to the chemicals from insulation and other materials in the motor and drive belt.

6. Joints in the galvanized sheet metal ducts are many times loosely fitted and sealed only by use of adhesive tape to prevent outside air intake, thus exposing the adhesive to the air stream in the ducts.

7. Dust filters are oiled to make them more effective.

8. Electrostatic filters, when used, not only produce ozone, a toxic material, but also produce odors from burned organic material related to arcing.

9. Some building codes require that an outside air intake be installed in the system.

10. When incitant chemicals arose within the living space or leaked in from outside, a long time was required to rid the air of the offending material.

With the foregoing considerations in mind, for my Gulf Coast location where minimum temperatures are seldom lower than 24°F to 26°F in winter and where hot weather is of seven-months duration, a conventional heat pump unit was chosen. This avoided the resistance electric or natural gas heating elements. In the heating phase of the heat pump, the heat exchange coils have a temperature range of 95°F to 120°F and produce no carbonizing of particulate matter in the air stream (Figure 16-1).

For clearing the air of incitant chemicals when they contaminated the air in the living space, a bank of activated charcoal

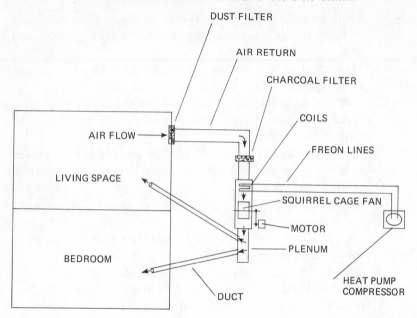

Figure 16-1. Modified central system for conditioning air.

was installed in the duct system.

To install a system of this sort that avoided the problems listed required much revision of usual methods and a cooperative air conditioning contractor. Even then, each step in installation required rigid supervision.

The galvanized sheet metal ducts were fabricated to provide a very tight fit at all joints. The tight fit was then maintained with tape on the outside. The tape was selected for having adhesive with very little odor. With the tight-fitting joints the adhesive of the tape was not exposed to the airstream inside the ducts.

No glue of any sort was used inside the duct system. All the insulation within the air return, plenum, and blower unit was 100 percent glass fiber with no plastic bonding. In the insulating trade this is called glass wool and the contractor obtained it by special order in rolls 36 to 48 inches wide and 100 feet long. Cut to desired size with shears, it was fastened in place with galvanized hardware cloth and sheet metal screws

(Figure 16-2). This insulation reduced air flow noise within the system as well as reducing heat loss or gain through the duct wall.

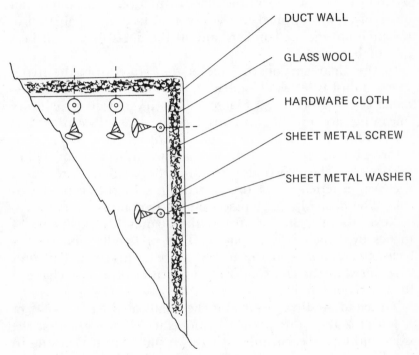

DUCT WALL

GLASS WOOL

HARDWARE CLOTH

SHEET METAL SCREW

SHEET METAL WASHER

Figure 16-2. Installation of glass wool within ducts.

The air handler (cooling-heating coils and blower) unit was remodeled to remove the sources of chemical incitants. The motor was removed and mounted on the outside of the unit. The shaft of the squirrel cage blower was replaced with one long enough to allow the drive pulley and belt to be placed outside the unit.

The drip pan was removed by cutting the framework of the air handler. It was then replaced with a pan fabricated of stainless steel by the sheet metal contractor. This avoided the need for a rust preventive.

The side and top panels of the air handler with their glued-on insulation were discarded and replaced with galvanized sheet metal panels to which the glass wool insulation was attached as described (Figure 16-2).

After the system was in place with all tight-fitting joints securely taped, ordinary fiberglass insulation with aluminum outer layer was applied to the outer surface of the air return, the plenum, the air handler, and all the ducts to prevent heat loss or heat gain.

In the airstream, on the side of the return from the living space, a dust filter was installed in the duct system. For maintenance convenience it was placed at floor level. A disposable, dry (meaning not oiled) paint-arrester-type glass-fiber filter was used. This was obtained by special order from a filter fabricator. This filtered dust from the air stream to prevent its impaction on the charcoal filter and the resultant premature decrease in efficiency of the charcoal in absorption of chemicals. The dust filter is replaced at least monthly.

Next, the activated charcoal filter banks (24 inches by 24 inches by 7 inches) were placed. The air handler size was selected to accommodate the air resistance of this filter. This unit is replaced as the charcoal becomes inefficient. It is exchanged for reactivated units.

To avoid air flow bypassing the charcoal filter, a gasket of 1/4 to 1/2 inch thick white orthopedic felt was used on the sides and top of each unit as it was installed in its housing in the duct. This increased the efficiency of the filter. It is the only gasket material I was able to find that did not contribute volatile chemicals to the air stream. This grade of orthopedic felt is very tightly packed and in its location was considered to contribute no particulate matter to the air stream.

Entrance of so-called fresh air from outside into the living space was avoided every way possible. There was enough air exchange by passage through doors to maintain sufficient oxygen supply. The circulation of the ambient air in the living quarters through the charcoal bank in the duct system kept it fresh smelling.

This living area has been carefully monitored by my most cooperative and helpful wife to avoid introduction of furnishings, clothing, cosmetics, and cleaning supplies that contribute chemicals to the air. Special attention was given to avoid introduction of materials that emanate chemicals at a level, or of a character, that has a noticeable odor. The television set and music system were located in cabinets in which small electric fans exhaust the chemicals produced by this electronic equipment through ducts from the cabinets to the outside.

During a major part of the time, the central system operates, either heating or cooling, and maintains a comfortable, fresh-smelling environment with a minimum of exposure to incitant chemicals.

When this central air treatment system was first put into operation with air being filtered by so large a volume of activated charcoal I was startled by the appearance of a "yeasty" odor in the air. Investigation led to the realization that it arose from the charcoal. I looked on the occurrence of this odor with such alarm that the charcoal filters were removed until I was able to determine what it meant. Considerable inquiry finally led to the work of Amos Turk, which suggested the "yeasty odor" sensation created when air was circulated through a large volume of activated charcoal was the manner in which the sense of smell records a complete or nearly complete absence of odor-producing chemicals from ambient air (1,2). With this consideration in mind, I have used this characteristic of activated charcoal to monitor its efficiency in absorbing chemicals. When circulation of the ambient air in my living quarters through the central air treatment systems fails to produce this "yeasty-odor" state, within twenty to thirty minutes (except when some chemical known to be particularly persistent has polluted the ambient air) I know it is time to replace the charcoal filters. I have also noted that when this "yeasty-odor" state exists in the ambient air, the introduction of any odor-producing chemical is more readily detected.

I have noted another consideration relating to detection of chemicals in the air by the sense of smell. When a chemical is introduced into the air in my living space and no circulation of the air through the charcoal filters is done, if I remain in the area, after five to ten minutes, my sense of smell ceases to register the odor of the chemical. If I then leave the area for five minutes or longer, on returning, I am again able to register the odor of the chemical. I have learned, therefore, that, as long as I remain in a given area, I cannot depend on my sense of smell to tell me when an odorous chemical pollutant has disappeared from the air.

This application of air treatment has not been without its limitations. Despite careful attention to avoiding leakage of outside air into the living space, there is still some small amount of outside air getting in. Because of the negative pressure in the air-return side of the duct system, this leakage is increased when the central system is in operation. Therefore, during periods of heavy concentration of pollutants in outside air, the central air treatment system is not operated. Instead, during cold periods electric hot water heaters are used to maintain comfortable temperatures. During hot weather, the uncomfortably warm temperatures in the living space are tolerated as the lesser of the two evils.

When the concentration of pollutants in outside air is extremely heavy, especially when winds are strong, there is leakage of a troublesome concentration of pollutant chemicals into the living space despite all these measures. During such periods I have used "personal" depollution of the contaminated air by use of a cannister-type activated charcoal respirator to avoid or minimize the troublesome exposure. Then, when the period of pollution has passed, I circulate the ambient air through the charcoal filters in the central system until the contaminating chemicals are removed and my "oasis" is again established.

I have applied this approach to central air treatment in my office space. This, along with a number of other measures, has made it possible for me to maintain an active medical practice.

The building was built specifically for my use in its entirety. Finishes and furnishings were selected to contribute the least possible chemical emanations to the air within the building. The autoclave was set to operate under an exhaust hood. All materials and supplies are selected for minimal chemical production. My staff uses only unscented cosmetics at work. Patients reporting for consultations are instructed to use only unscented or no cosmetics on the day of consultation. Thus, they bring with them a minimum of perfume from the previous day's use in clothing or hair. The constant circulation of ambient air through the charcoal filter in the air treatment system further reduces the amount of perfume and other chemical incitants in the air to a level that, with the use of large size personal activated charcoal respirator under my desk, allows me to keep my exposure to these incitants within the bounds of tolerance most of the time.

For the benefit of the small number of my patients who are hypersensitive to chemicals, their visits are scheduled for times when it is least likely that other patients will introduce perfumes into the ambient air.

"PERSONAL" TREATMENT OF AIR

Activated charcoal has been used many years in *respirators* in military and industrial applications for protection of individuals from toxic chemicals. The objective of this use was reduction of the concentration of the material to a level that short-term exposure of a person would not produce poisoning — thus, the military or industrial gas mask.

In the person with chemical hypersensitivity, exposure to even small concentrations of his incitants produces troublesome reaction. Reduction of concentration of the exposure by use of a charcoal respirator reduces the severity of the reaction. The lower the concentration of chemicals in ambient air and the larger the bed of activated charcoal to pull it through, the more near 100 percent removal of the chemicals from the air on one passage through the charcoal will be and, consequently, the lower the level of exposure of the individual using the respirator will be. This, of course, is the impetus behind efforts to reduce the level of chemical incitants in the ambient air in which a person places himself and behind the use of a personal charcoal respirator.

The ordinary industrial gas mask cannister contains approximately one pound of fine particle-size charcoal, which was inadequate for my use. I designed and had fabricated from stainless steel sheet metal a cannister that holds 3.5 pounds of charcoal to be used with a portable respirator. This is of a size that can be carried on a shoulder strap, much as a large ladies' handbag is carried. The loaded cannister weighs about 7 pounds. One passage of air through this volume of charcoal will remove all or nearly all of low-level concentrations of many chemicals. The portable respirator, thus, allows me to meet some circumstances of chemically contaminated air with much less or no reaction and allows a somewhat greater mobility. During periods of heavy air pollution when some chemicals seep into my living quarters despite closed doors and windows, use of the portable respirator provides most helpful protection. Unfortunately, though, the concentrations of incitants in the ambient air of most shops and other public places is so high that passage of the air through the portable respirator does not sufficiently remove troublesome chemicals from the air. Also, the level of perfume concentration in ambient air built up in a small room from even one person who has put on perfume, cologne, after-shave lotion, hairspray, hair dressing, deodorants, or any number of other scented preparations during the previous twelve to fifteen hours is so great that one passage of air through the portable respirator still leaves a troublesome concentration of contamination in the air. Use of the respirator, therefore, does not allow close contact with many patients in ordinary clinic situations without troublesome exposure.

For the above reason I designed and had fabricated from galvanized sheet metal a large cannister (Figure 16-3). This unit, which sits under my desk in my consultation room, holds approximately 25 pounds of activated charcoal, and when loaded, weighs approximately 40 pounds. By the baffle arrangement, the air flows through a column of charcoal 3 inches by 5 inches by 10 feet long. This charcoal bed will filter out 100 percent of moderate to heavy concentrations of most perfume on one passage through it. Even use of this large cannister respirator has its limitations. There are certain perfumes that, even with so large an amount of charcoal, require many passages through the cannister for complete removal of the odor. Also, with even moderate concentrations of perfume, there is a very small movement of perfume-laden air into the nasal cavity when I talk while using the respirator. To prevent a problem from arising from this exposure in such circumstances, I must put on my nose a clip of a sort that some swimmers use.

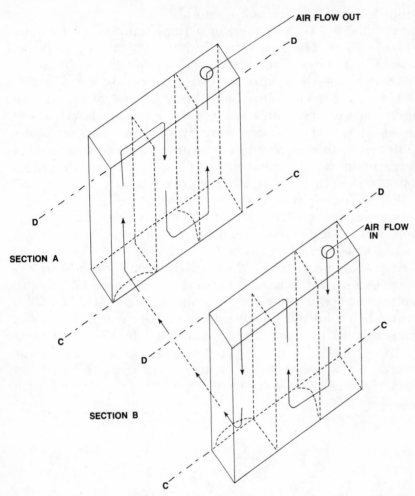

AIR FLOW OUT

D

C

D

D

AIR FLOW IN

SECTION A

C

C

D

D

SECTION B

C

Figure 16-3. Large cannister. Section A and Section B joined at D-D, C-C.

The charcoal in each of these cannisters is replaced periodically, as its effectiveness indicates. This varies according to the level of pollutants in the air in which the respirator is used.

To provide a mouth bit and a flexible airway that would allow for use of these cannisters without imparting chemical contamination to the airstream posed quite a problem. Every mouthpiece investigated was constructed of rubber and/or plastic, and no matter how old the structural material, it continued to emanate incitant chemicals.

The mouth bit was fabricated from stainless steel tubing (Figure 16-4). The airway was fashioned after the manner of many air ducts — a coil of wire with a fabric cover (Figure 16-5). Small gauge galvanized steel wire was closely wound onto a 1 1/4 inch diameter pipe. This, then, was stretched to give an evenly spaced coil with the wire coils approximately 1/8 inch apart. It was then washed with Ivory® soap and hot water followed by thorough rinsing to remove incitant chemicals that were on the wire. One end of the coil was fastened to the mouth bit and the other end to the cannister fitting.

For the cannister end, the fittings for fastening an industrial gas mask airway to the cannister were salvaged. The male fitting was fabricated into the charcoal cannister. The galvanized wire coil was fastened to the female fitting.

It was found that the thin polyethylene film used by dry cleaners for clothes bags, if allowed to air for several months, appeared to cease emanating incitant chemicals. This polyfilm was rolled onto the galvanized coils to five or six thicknesses and fastened in place in its mid-portion by ties of strips of polyfilm. At each end it was fastened to the metal tubing, the mouth bit at one end and the female fitting at the other, by masking tape. Care was taken to apply the tape to only that

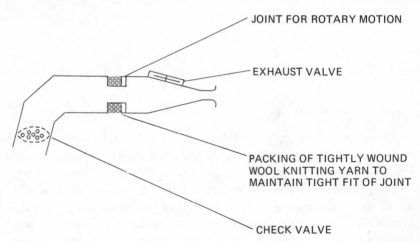

JOINT FOR ROTARY MOTION

EXHAUST VALVE

PACKING OF TIGHTLY WOUND WOOL KNITTING YARN TO MAINTAIN TIGHT FIT OF JOINT

CHECK VALVE

Figure 16-4. Mouth bit, longitudinal cross section.

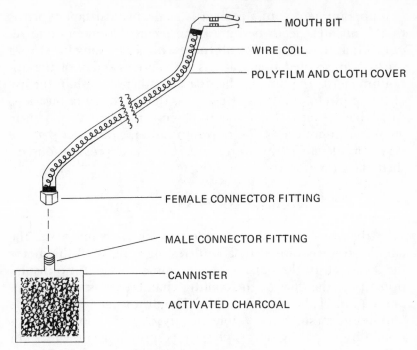

Figure 16-5. Airway.

portion of the film that overlaid the metal tubing, so no incitants from the adhesive would be imparted to the air stream. A cloth cover was sewed in place to protect the plastic film and give it a better appearance. Periodically during use, the polyfilm and cloth cover are replaced. If it were available, I feel that a cellophane film of a sort used in food packaging would serve very well instead of the polyfilm.

There are times when a patient becomes acutely ill, e.g. has an acute asthma attack, and must come in for consultation without being able to plan for the visit. On these occasions by use of this large cannister respirator and a nose clip, it is possible for me to talk to and examine the patient and still avoid a bad reaction to the perfume or other chemicals he may bring with him.

"What," you may ask, "is the attitude of a patient to a grotesque figure behind a desk with a breathing apparatus in his mouth and, at times, a clip on his nose?" At the time when the first appointment with a patient is made, my assistant explains that I am allergic to perfumes and scented cosmetics and requests that the patient and all those who accompany him avoid use of any scented preparations on the entire day of the appointment. At the time of the first visit, then, I explain the use of the respirator, and why I use it, as the first order of business. After that, as far as I am able to observe, the patients pay little attention to my use of the respirator and for the most part are very considerate in avoiding use of scented preparations on their days for reserved appointments.

WINDOW AIR CONDITIONERS

In the type of window unit I have used in my oasis, the circulated air is moved by a squirrel cage fan, with the motor for it located in the outside of the cabinet. There is no insulation inside the duct or the cooling chamber to assure no contamination of the air (Fig. 16-6). The dust filter I have used is aluminum mesh. Since I tolerate *glycerin* of coconut derivation, a light coating of this glycerin is sprayed over the mesh in order to increase the efficiency of dust collection. The filter is washed periodically with mild soap solution, and after having been dried thoroughly, the filter mesh is again treated with glycerin.

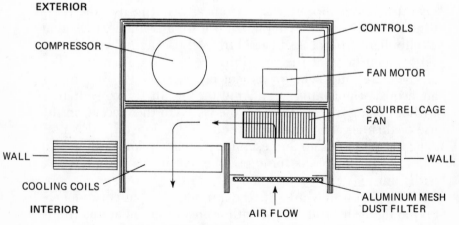

Figure 16-6. Window air conditioner unit.

SUMMARY

The use of an oasis and the portable charcoal respirator has made it possible for me to spend several hours each day in a clinic setting. The cooperative staff uses only lightly scented cosmetics, and the patients scheduled for appointments with me are instructed to use no scented cosmetics on the day of the appointment. Furnishings, finishes, and the supplies that are used in the clinic have been chosen to assure minimum chemical incitation. Activated charcoal filters are used in the central air conditioning system, which is equipped with steam coils for heating the air, when necessary.

A small office has been set aside for my personal isolation in case of emergency developments. Furnishings in this office have been selected to provide maximum freedom from chemical outgassing. The room is completely separated from the clinic's air treatment system. The window air conditioner keeps my isolation room cool. For heating, an electric hot water heater has been installed to keep me comfortable.

When perfume or other chemical contamination occurs in the clinic's central air conditioning system in a concentration too great for my tolerance despite the assistance of my portable charcoal respirator, I retire to my oasis until the problem subsides.

All of these arrangements have required much effort and attention. It also has necessitated a major investment normally not required for a medical facility. But this afforded me the means of maintaining my medical practice, which is my means of survival.

Perhaps this recitation will be of some value by suggesting means for the improvement and the management of the indoor environment for other individuals who are hypersensitive to chemical contaminants. Despite the suggestion to be derived from the foregoing report, it would be well for each individual to experience a trial exposure to each of the materials intended for his specific environment. Such trial exposures would assure that the individual differences of chemical susceptibility would be appropriately provided for and that no major investments were made in error due to incorrect assumptions.

BIBLIOGRAPHY

1. Turk, Amos and Bownes, Kenneth: Inadequate stimulation of olfaction, *Science, 114* (2957): 234-236.
2. Smith, S.B.: Personal Communication, January 16, 1963.

Detailed specifications and drawings of the mouth bit, airway, and each of the cannisters, as well as the charcoal respirator and the various sources of materials, may be obtained from the author. Address: P.O. Box 3038, Port Arthur, TX 77640.

Chapter 17

GUIDELINES FOR AN ECOLOGIC AIR CONDITIONING SYSTEM

SIDNEY J. HEIMAN

AIR conditioning, as it is commonly referred to, is actually only air cooling. This method of treating air for comfort purposes has become a way of life for many people in our society. In some areas of our country, air conditioning is a necessity, especially in many work situations. To be compatible for the hypersensitive individual, many variations from the usual installation of air conditioning must be considered. The following ten observations will assure the development of a more tolerable air conditioning system for the hypersensitive individual:

1. Low velocity of air exchange is imperative. The tactile sensation of a draft or feeling of air movement can often produce illness in the individual who is afflicted with what is sometimes referred to as "thermal allergy."
2. Oversized air ducts and grills help. This tends to decrease both the air pressure and the air velocity. The result is minimum ambient air disturbance, thus, lesser stirring of ambient microscopic particulates.
3. Provide a constant flow of air at median temperature. This is more tolerable to the hypersensitive individual than extreme temperatures supplied at shorter and irregular intervals.
4. A broad spectrum of filtration is mandatory. This type of air depollution must remove gaseous contaminants from the occupied space, as well as most of the microscopic particulates, and not produce ozone as a by-product.
5. The motors and fans must be isolated. To accomplish this the moving machinery should be installed outside the air-cooling box. The patient should monitor the in-

159

stallation carefully to assure that no motor is installed inside the box.

6. Removal of moisture is important. The drainage of the collected moisture is especially important. Stagnation of improperly drained moisture may provide a media for mold growth and consequent illness to the hypersensitive person.

7. Individual room units may be preferred. Zoned control is more easily achieved this way. Cross-contamination of ambient odors between various rooms can be controlled better with the individual room units.

8. Mechanical filtration of the conditioned air is generally inadequate. At best, it removes only larger particulates but fails to remove gases and odors.

9. Outside air input is undesirable. The usual structural leakage and air intake through doors, at time of entrance and exit incidents, is sufficient. If outside air input is necessary, then it should be filtered at the point of intake.

10. Install the compressor unit outside. Although incipient leakage of refrigerant gases is rare, its hazard is too great to risk an inside installation of the compressor unit.

The foregoing is provided as an alert to the design engineer, whose responsibility will be to provide a hypersensitive individual with a compatible air-cooling system. Various approaches can be made to condition the air of the occupied space; however, the ultimate should meet the above minimum standards.

Appendices

Appendix A

TAX COMMENTARY

D. B. WARNOCK

THE preceding chapters of this book deal
with the various medical and structural problems arising from
exposure to pollution or other environmental irritants. They
show how you can overcome or reduce your sensitivity to the
environmental influences, how you can become more efficient
thereby, how to become more energetic and comfortable in
spite of them, and how you can eliminate the most offensive
pollutants from your home.

To accomplish the recommended developments involves a
major financial outlay. There are many unusual medical expenses involved, as well as the expense of special equipment for
heating, cooking, or air conditioning when prescribed. Many
such costs may be considerably reduced if you know how to use
the medical-deduction portion of your income tax report form.
To obtain full value of the various medical deductions, it is
necessary to consider several things: (1) you need to know what
the deductible expenditures are, how to list them, and how to
prove them; (2) you need to obtain the necessary proofs for
these deductions; (3) you need the help of a professional tax
attorney or a qualified certified public accountant (CPA).

In this monograph we assume that you know there is no
point in itemizing your deductions unless they exceed the
amount of the current standard medical deduction allowed. We
also assume that you know that home remedies and commonly
used items, such as aspirin, patent medicines, toothpaste, and
other sanitizing preparations, are considered personal comfort
items and are not deductible unless they are prescribed by a
physician. It is also assumed that you accept the word "physician" as used in this discussion, which means any person or
group of such persons who are skilled in the medical healing
arts and who are duly licensed to practice under your state laws.

CLASS I TAX-DEDUCTIBLE ITEMS

The broad general rule for all medical deductions is that you may deduct the cost of any expenses that can be proven as necessary to improve or to maintain your health. First of all this includes specific medical expenses prescribed by your physician: (1) appliances and their upkeep — repairs — cost of their operation, ambulance services, artificial limbs, dental services and cost of dentures; (2) eye examinations and eyeglasses; (3) acupuncture; (4) all medical examination fees; (5) all hospitalization fees, such as oxygen tent rental, costs for oxygen used (including pickup and delivery charges), syringes, hospitalization insurance premiums, nurses' fees, surgical and obstetrical charges, and other special treatments; (6) Seeing Eye® dogs, their training, food, and upkeep; and (7) transportation costs, telephone charges (including the cost of voice amplifiers), and many other costs that are too numerous to list here or that may vary from time to time. The list of such tax-deductible items increases some years and decreases in other years. In order to obtain full deductions it is necessary to ascertain the current items and their limitations each year.

CLASS II TAX-DEDUCTIBLE ITEMS

You may deduct other various expenses that promote health, even though you may not think of them as medical in nature. These items include such things as the cost of removing furnaces, water heaters, stoves, and gas lines, as well as the cost of their replacement with electrical devices or appliances. These deductible items also include costs for additional electrical circuits, heavier wiring, additional bath facilities, and any structural changes in your home or in its furnishings — if they are performed on the specific orders of your physician in writing.

The travel expenses that you may deduct include the cost of the round trip to your physician's office, if he is located out of your home town, as well as transportation of the patient to the hospital. Such out-of-town travel includes mileage, meals and lodging, if required, which are also added to deductions. The law makes no limitation on the distance you travel to consult the physician of your choice, but it does require that you travel by the shortest distance or over the most direct route. If your condition requires that you be accompanied by a nurse or by some other skilled person in medical treatments, the cost of such an escort is deductible including his/her meals and lodging.

In many families several members contribute to the support of a parent or of another member of the family in amounts that gives no contributor over one-half of the total support. In such cases the personal tax exemption of the party supported should be given to whatever person in the group will benefit most by the added medical expense and by the personal deduction of the party so supported. In such cases it is best to make a special bank account into which all contributions are deposited and all checks for support items drawn. Multiple support forms must be filed with the return of the party taking the exemption.

The deduction for the extra cost of diets is very tricky. The rules are often changed, but the broad general rule is that the diet must not replace ordinary food the average person consumes. If you include such cost among your deductions, include or attach a statement from your physician that such items are prescribed solely for the alleviation or treatment of your existing illness.

All deductions for medical expense must show that the item or items are additional medical expenses and not expenses that would not have been incurred had the medical necessity not been established.

CLASS III, PROOF FOR TAX DEDUCTIONS

All medical deductions must be proven. You will need a receipt from your druggist showing the date, prescription number, and the amount paid for each prescription. You will need a copy of the prescriptions for all medical equipment, appliances, and home changes, and receipts for the same, as well as for travel expenses paid by you. The physician's statement should show the specific illness or malfunction from which you are suffering and the necessity of the items he prescribes; for example, reference to the items required to remodel your home for the purpose of improving your health or to keep it from deteriorating should be included.

Where home improvements are required, you will also need the written statement from an established real estate agent showing what portion of the change in the home, if any, increases the monetary value of your property. If the property is made more valuable by the change, the added value becomes a part of the cost of your property and can only be recovered at the time of its sale. In the case of improvements to rental property, the increased value must be divided by the remaining time your lease has to run and is deducted annually over the unexpired life of your lease. It is also worth noting that the cost of the real estate appraisal can be deducted as a miscellaneous tax-deductible item in your return, and it should be shown as an appraisal fee in the last paragraph of the deduction sheet listing.

Except for drugs purchased (which may be entered as a single figure) copies of all proofs of payment, or receipts, should be stapled to the tax return. The originals of the payment records should be kept at least seven years for future reference. If you have more than one hospitalization insurance policy (including such amount in your automobile policy), the total cost of such hospitalization insurance may be entered as one figure. If you are on medicare, be sure to add the coinsurance charges to your hospital item.

EXAMPLES OF MEDICAL DEDUCTIONS UNDER
THE PRECEDING RULES

There are three types of expenditures: (1) those that increase the value of the home; (2) those that do not increase the value of the home; and (3) those that increase the cost of home construction over standard costs involved in the same type of construction. To illustrate these principles the following examples are included:

1. This example involves the installation of a first-floor bath with toilet and bowl. This expenditure has been prescribed by your physician in writing because your physical condition at

the time and in the future requires you to make this structural change in your home. This change in your residence will usually increase its value to some extent. The tax revenue agent will argue that the entire cost of the remodeling is the measure of the increased value of your home — that you must add it to the value of your home and recover it when you sell the property. In order to recover a fair proportion of the expenditure, it is necessary to have a real estate agent give you the amount, if any, that such installation increases the value of your home. The difference in the amount expended and the increased value of the property is the amount you are entitled to deduct as a medical expense. Should any item ordered to be installed cost more than the usual standard item, the statement should prescribe the more costly item and the advantages derived in its value.

2. An example of a prescribed change that would not increase the value of your residence would be the replacement of drapes, eliminating the chemical property of the material you are sensitive to. The same is true of some paints, but here the cost is greater because the old paint must be removed and be replaced with a new formula that gives you no harmful reaction. Assuming the troublesome paint was recently installed, neither expenditure increases the value of the premises.

3. In this example we deal with the increased cost of construction of your residence over the standard construction costs, which raises a great number of questions. In such matters your builder may have to submit to you figures showing the excess cost over the cost of usual and standard construction. Such costs can start with the footings of the building, the structural materials, adhesives, other chemical and synthetic materials, and insulating materials, even to the installation of a hard-topped driveway, which may require substitution of asphalt with concrete. It is very possible that in the future the tax revenue department will require such proofs in remodeling matters, also.

The installation of a central air conditioning system illustrates a mixture of costs exemplified under the first and third listing previously mentioned. The tax revenue agent will argue that the entire cost increases the value of your home. You meet this argument by showing that the bedroom is used only part of the day, whereas, the entire living quarters of the house are used the greater part of the day. At present the prescription of your physician and a real estate appraisal will eliminate this objection, but do not be surprised if, in the future, you need a statement from your contractor showing the amount of the increase in cost where such an appliance is installed.

INTERNAL REVENUE SERVICE
QUESTIONS OF CLAIMS

If tax-deductible items are of value to you, remember that a job worth doing is worth doing well. This suggests the last matter to which you should give serious thought — namely, the employment of a tax expert who has your personal interest foremost in his mind and who will take the time to go over your deductions at length with you. In making such a selection, remember that under existing law only licensed attorneys and certified public accountants can go with you and are permitted to represent you legally in all matters and questions that may arise should your return be audited by the Internal Revenue Service (IRS). All other tax preparation persons can only state what you told them to include in your tax return.

The legal tax expert can help you word your items so that they are presented appropriately in your return. This often makes the difference in acceptance or rejection of an item.

Should you decide to work out your own return, secure and study carefully government pamphlets on the subject of medical deductions. There are many other tax guides including paperback books, but the list is too long to be set out here.

In all tax matters, remember that to obtain deductions you must apply for them. If you do not enter deductions on your return, the revenue service will not do it for you, even if you are entitled to such a deduction. Generally speaking, it is better to enter and take a chance on the revenue service rejecting a questionable item than it is for you to omit claiming it on your return. This is true even though there may be a number of such items. It may be three years before your return is audited; in the meantime the law and the rulings of the tax service may make these deductions acceptable.

At this point you are cautioned that in all tax audits, when a question is presented it must be thoroughly understood before you answer. Take your time in answering. If you are in doubt, ask the examiner to restate the question. An innocent-sounding question may not call for the answer you think of first. Never volunteer personal opinion. Should you become convinced that the examiner is unfriendly or is not treating you fairly, end the interview and ask the supervisor of the examiner's division (which may be a field office or an audit division) to assign your audit to another person. Should you decide that the final assessment made by an examiner is unfair, do not hesitate to appeal the examiner's findings.

SUMMARY

1. Know your deductions and their limitations.

2. Obtain written statements that justify your deductions. These should be obtained from your physicians, your hospital, your pharmacist, your real estate agent, and/or building contractor.

3. Document all costs and expenses pertaining to your deductions, especially thost that may improve your property.

4. Keep and preserve all documents seven years.

Appendix B

MATTRESS ECOLOGY

CASIMIR M. NIKEL

EARLY in the historical development of clinical ecology it was known that the mattress was highly offensive to individuals with house dust sensitivity. To combat this problem mattresses were often encased in plastic covers. This eventually was proven to be a mistake. Individuals with chemical susceptibility were exchanging a lesser evil for a greater one by the use of synthetic mattress covers.

The problem with synthetic materials for mattress ticking has been complicated since May 31, 1972, because of legal implications. At that time the United States Department of Commerce issued a mandatory regulation that all mattresses manufactured after twelve months from the date of that notice must be flame proofed. The regulation in question is titled "Flammability Standard For Mattresses (DOC FF 4-72)."

The mattress materials usable under DOC FF 4-72 are intolerable to individuals with chemical susceptibility. At first the development imposed by DOC FF 4-72 was met with consternation in clinical ecology circles. The regulation was found to be complex and lengthy. It indicated thirty exclusions; however, none of them seemed to apply to a conventional mattress used on the beds for adults. Despite its limited scope, it seemed that the door was closed to custom fabrication of mattresses under the definition set forth in Section .2-(a) of the regulation. The definition reads as follows: "Mattress means a ticking filled with a resilient material used alone or in combination with other products and intended or promoted for sleeping upon. This definition includes, but is not limited to, mattress pads, adult mattresses, youth mattresses, crib mattresses including portable crib mattresses, bunk bed mattresses, convertible sofa bed mattresses, corner group mattresses, day bed mattresses, rollaway bed mattresses, high-risers, and trundle bed mattresses."

Based on the foregoing definition of a mattress, and under the specific requirements that such mattresses meet the standard of nonflammability, it is not permissible for a manufacturer to construct a conventional mattress for a hypersensitive individual from cotton material untreated with flame-resisting chemicals. Careful examination, however, of DOC FF 4-72 reveals the following in Section .2-(d): "One of a kind mattress, such as non standard sizes or shapes, may be excluded from testing under this standard pursuant to rules and regulations established by the Federal Trade Commission." It seems, therefore, that the exclusion of mattresses slightly larger or slightly smaller and those that are "one of a kind" opens the door for a manufacturer to fabricate a custom-made mattress for a hypersensitive individual to the specifications of the patient.

It is suggested, therefore, that an individual with chemical susceptibility contact a local mattress factory and negotiate for the fabrication of a mattress under the provision indicated previously. If your local manufacturer does not have a copy of DOC FF 4-72, it can be obtained directly from the United States Department of Commerce in Washington, D.C.

After an agreement for custom fabrication of a mattress from natural cotton materials is achieved, the hypersensitive individual must provide the manufacturer with the specifications tolerable to him. This may be difficult for one undergoing such an experience for the first time. Some suggestions, therefore are provided.

Specifications for a custom-built mattress under the exclusion listed in DOC FF 4-72 .2-(d):

1. Size should be two inches shorter than standard in the trade.
2. Core of the mattress should be of coil springs, and they should be tied together, preferably with wire.
3. Edging of the core must be padded with cotton felt, but be sure that the felt is not treated with flame-proofing chemicals.
4. The top and bottom surface of the core is to be padded with quilted cotton. Again, be sure that it is untreated with fire-proofing chemicals. The quilted pad should be

laundered by the customer to eliminate sizing, which often is troublesome to the hypersensitive individual.

5. The outermost layer, which is termed "ticking," must be of cotton material. It also must not be treated with flame-proofing chemicals, and it should be laundered by the customer before it is used by the manufacturer for fabrication of the mattress.

6. The material used for taping the edges of the mattress on the outside of the ticking must be cotton, and the same exclusion of flame proofing applies as above. Also, laundering before fabrication is preferred if the fabricator can use limp tape.

7. Be sure to emphasize in your request that the ticking not be pierced for installation of buttons. Omit the buttons. This technique is used to give the mattress a smooth appearance; however, this is troublesome to the hypersensitive individual. The cotton felt inside of the mattress tends to produce dust, which is pumped to the outside. The pumping effect is created by the restless movements of the sleeping person.

More often than not when the customer arrives to pick up his mattress, he discovers that specification number seven has been overlooked. This is due mostly to the pride of workmanship. It is impossible to stretch laundered ticking so a trim and smooth appearance is achieved. The craftsman in the factory may decide against original instructions not to button down the mattress surfaces, thinking that the customer would not accept the wrinkly and untidy-looking mattress.

Should this happen to you, do not be upset. Recognize the good intention of the workman and resort to a remedial technique. Purchase a quilted cotton pad and use it under the sheet. If you purchase a standard-size pad, it is long enough to overhang the top end of the mattress, which tends to direct downward microscopic dust particles that are pumped outward around the buttons. This overhang of the pad directs the dust away from your face and minimizes the possibility of dust reaction.

The outer quilted pad provides another service besides preventing dust from reaching your nostrils. Body heat and moisture tend to spawn mold growth in bedding fabrics. The quilted pad can be laundered, thereby providing a protection not otherwise achieved. The frequency of laundering of the pad can be determined by observing troublesome symptoms, particularly nasal blockage during the night.

The foregoing information is obviously brief and generalized. The mattress ecology is more complex than this discussion implies. It is hopefully a pointer, however, in the right direction for those who may have been unaware of the exclusion in Section .2-(d) of the Document FF 4-72 and its potential for permitting custom fabrication of mattresses for the chemically susceptible individual.

Appendix C

FINISHING MATERIALS

GUY O PFEIFFER

A MAJOR troublesome group of materials for developing the ecologic house can be paints, varnishes, shellacs, and other finishing products. Some of these finishing materials have been known to outgas for several years. It is imperative, therefore, that the chemically susceptible individual be tested for tolerance to a specific brand and to the specific production lot of a specific brand of finishing material before it is considered safe to use in the space to be occupied by the hypersensitive person.

The finishing materials consist of several substances, such as the vehicle, the drying agent, the pigment, pesticides, and fungicides. Any one of these substances may prove to be troublesome to the hypersensitive individual. The variety of formulations for finishing materials is legion, and it undergoes continual modifications. Consequently, no specific type or brand of paint, varnish, or shellac can be recommended.

To assist the reader in this respect, the following guidelines are suggested:

1. Secure a small quantity of a finishing product desired. Cover a scrap of plasterboard, or a piece of lumber with it, and allow ample drying time for the fumes to outgas.
2. Perform the sniff test by smelling the test piece for several minutes at frequent intervals, until you are satisfied that the product is acceptable or unacceptable to the chemically susceptible individual.

The use of shellac is often acceptable. In spite of the fact that it is dissolved in hydrocarbon alcohol, after it is applied to the woodwork, the outgassing is usually complete within several weeks. It is not as durable as varnish and other similar products. Also, it is susceptible to being dissolved by spilled alcoholic drinks on tables and other flat surfaces.

174

Some types of alkyd paints have been observed to be tolerable by some individuals. Water-based paints must be evaluated with great caution due to such additives as pesticides and fungicides.

Varnish and synthetic substitutes must be evaluated by individual brand and by the individual production lot number.

Testing of individual products is slow and time consuming. The potential hazard of using an intolerable material for finishing the inside of the house designed for chemically susceptible persons, however, is too great to risk not testing the paints first. The sniff test therefore is strongly urged. Where it is feasible, the tactile sensitivity test might be applied. For fuller information on the latter form of testing, the reader is referred to Chapter 45 of *Clinical Ecology* (1).

One authority suggests that caution be used in repainting, despite tested tolerance to a given finishing product, and especially with a seemingly tolerated paint sample (2). The concentration of outgassing by a small test sample may be insufficient to precipitate a reaction. A full house of the same material may outgas sufficiently to overwhelm the hypersensitive individual's level of tolerance. It is suggested, therefore, that a repainting of the house be done one room at a time. This gradual approach should especially start with rooms that the hypersensitive individual can avoid, should this prove to be necessary. However, by the time a couple of bedrooms are repainted with no perceptible reaction showing, it is presumably safe to proceed with the repainting of the larger living areas with the tested paint.

REFERENCES

1. Dickey, Lawrence D. (Ed.): *Clinical Ecology.* Springfield, Thomas, 1976.
2. Silver, Francis: Personal communication to the editors of this book.

GLOSSARY

A.C.E. Designation for "ambient chemical extraction" type of air purifiers. One such unit is available through the Depollution Division of the Air Conditioning Engineers at Decatur, Illinois.

ALLERGIES. Clinical ecologists use this term in a generic sense, which means that it includes reactions to allergens without demonstrating antibodies.

AMBIENT. This term has developed an uncertain connotation. In this book it refers to the surrounding space, regardless of its relation to the outdoor or indoor relationship.

CHEMICAL EXPOSURES. In clinical ecology this specifically refers to pollution contact with gaseous substances.

CHEMICAL SUSCEPTIBILITY. This designates senstivity to gaseous substances.

CLINICAL ECOLOGY. This branch of medicine is concerned with the process of adverse reactions from environmental insults to the human body and the consequent reactions and adaptation to such insults by the susceptible individual.

CLINICAL MANIFESTATIONS. Symptoms observed in individual patients during actual medical diagnostic or treatment procedures.

ECOLOGIC CLINICIANS. Specific reference to a physician practicing clinical ecology.

ECOLOGIC DISEASE. Reference to an ailment specifically caused by an environmental impact.

ECOLOGIC HOUSE. In this book this term is specifically designating a house that has been purged of incitants harmful to a chemically susceptible individual.

EMPIRICAL. Reference to tests or experiments from which the results are physically and numerically identifiable and that are capable of replication.

ENVIRONMENTAL CONSULTANT. A newly developing physician's aide trained to recognize unhealthful indoor ecologic conditions.

FRIED DUST. Specific term referring to house dust that has been carbonized by coming in contact with a heat exchanger in a furnace heated in excess of 300°F.

GLYCERIN. For individuals intolerant to coconut-derived glycerin, there is also a pork-derived glycerin. Also, whale oil, cottonseed oil, and similar vegetable oils are potential filter-spraying materials to be used by hypersensitive individuals.

GLYPTAL®. A trademark designation of an alkyd resin used to cover electrical

177

circuits such as motor windings.

HOPI RUGS. Rugs made by Indians of the Hopi tribe in western New Mexico.

HOT WATER HEATER. Refers specifically to a space heater manufactured by the Intertherm Company. This is a space heater and not a heater for increasing temperature in process water.

HOUSE-CALL CONSULTANT. Another term for environmental consultant.

HYPERSENSITIVITY. This is a generic term used in this book to designate individuals who are not only allergic in the classical sense but also who are responsive to chemicals that do not produce antibodies.

HYPOALLERGENIC. This term has been developed by commercial interests and is used generally to refer to items that produce none or a low level of allergic reaction in the hypersensitive individual.

INCITANTS. Any class of substances, precipitating illness in a hypersensitive individual, that consist of foods, pollens, molds, and/or gaseous chemicals.

INTERTHERM®. Trade name designation of an electrical hot water space heater.

LAMINAR INDUCTION. Process consisting of introducing air into a room through jet outlets at a low velocity. The jet outlets are spaced in such a way as to allow the air to move in equally arranged layers. This results in uniform thermal distribution.

OASIS. In this book this specifically refers to an isolated indoor space, such as one room within a residence, which has been decontaminated of harmful chemicals to the hypersensitive individual.

OUTGASSING. Molecular emanation from organic materials, such as petrochemical synthetic fabrics.

PLASTICIZERS. Chemicals that are used by the synthetic plastic manufacturers to give sheet plastics a flexible quality.

PNEUMOCONIOSIS. A condition of the respiratory tract due to inhalation of dust.

POLLUTION. Any substance or condition in the environment that harms the health of a human being. (It is recognized that some substances and conditions harmful to humans may be beneficial to other forms of life; therefore, this term in clinical ecology is restricted to the foregoing definition.)

PSYCHOTHERAPY. This term is used in a generic sense, indicating an effect on the total well-being of a hypersensitive individual. It does not refer to any specific psychiatric treatment methodology.

PURAFIL®. Trade name for an air-cleaning material.

RAYON. Currently, it is a material made of synthetic fibers; therefore, in the context of this book rayons must be considered as only those that are derived from wood or similar cellular substances.

RESISTANCE ELECTRIC HEATING. A direct application of heat through a coil or cable in a baseboard unit, which is done at high temperature resulting in fried dust. This is not the same as the recommended Intertherm.

RESPIRATOR. A similar personal depollution unit is commercially available from the Air Conditioning Engineers of Decatur, Illinois.

Sizing. Chemical substances that are used for filling and for stiffening fabrics.

Structural Respiration. The infiltration of outside air into a building through unplanned pathways, through wall cracks, around doors and windows, etc.

Terpenes. Hydrocarbon juices and fumes produced principally by evergreen trees.

Terpene Woods. This refers to conifer trees, which are a rich source of hydrocarbon oils, resins and fumes.

Thermal Pollution. Caused principally by high temperatures of such heating systems as forced air furnaces, resistance electric heaters, light bulbs, etc.

Ticking. Technical term for fabric used by upholsterers, principally for covering mattresses.

TV. Television sets and other high frequency equipment has been reported recently to have been recognized as harmful to hypersensitive individuals. This is probably due to heat, ozone, and microwave emanations. This is indicated here for those who may have reason to suspect such equipment.

Withdrawal Symptoms. This concept is generally associated with narcotic addiction. Clinical ecology has established that similar manifestations occur when a chemically susceptible individual discontinues exposures to a food or inhalant. In this book withdrawal symptoms refer exclusively to nonnarcotic addiction.

INDEX